SO GOOD

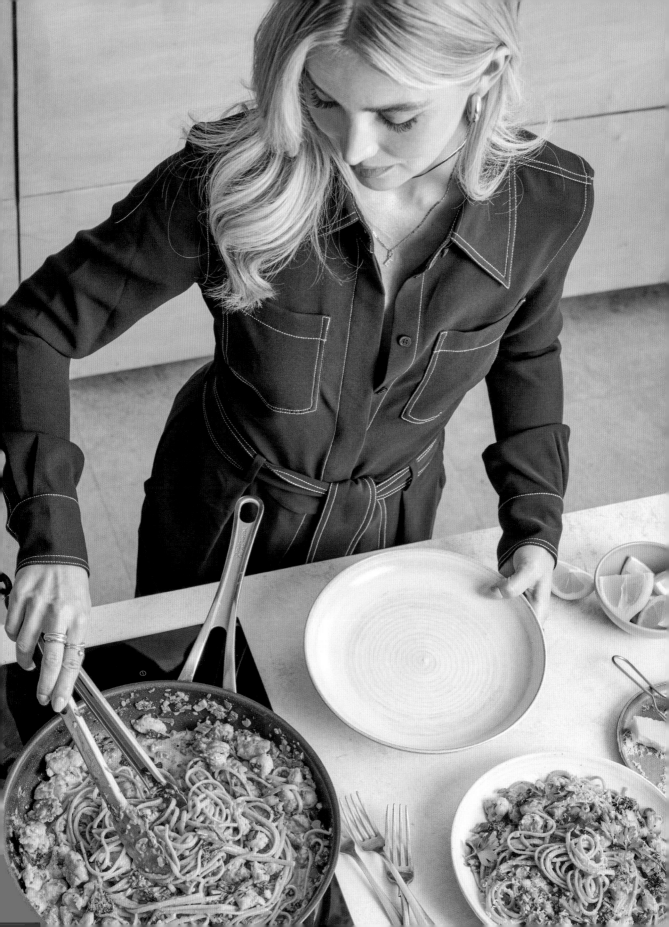

Food you want to eat,
designed by a nutritionist

SO GOOD

EMILY ENGLISH

SEVEN DIALS

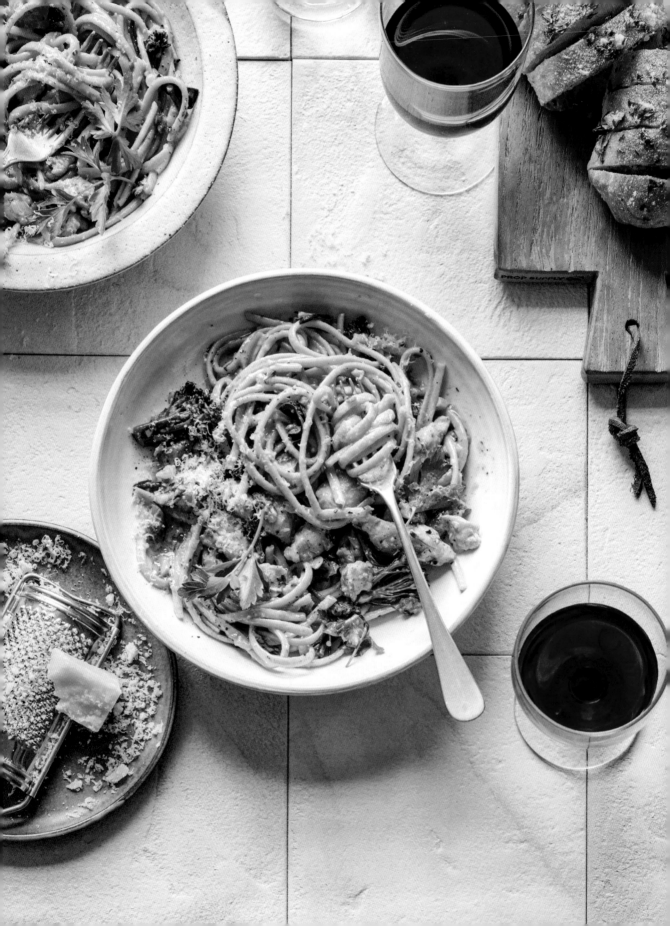

Introduction

vii

Breakfast

01

Lunch

41

Snacks

83

Dinner

97

Sweet

167

Meal Plans

193

Index & Conversions

203

Acknowledgements

212

Hello

Hello

Hello

My Journey to Joy

For most, a nutritionist would be the last person you want at your dream dinner party. Nutrition has been built up over the years to focus on rules around food, fearmongering and guilt. There is more misinformation out there than ever before, with a new clickbait headline every week or a social media fanatic analysing food on the supermarket shelves. So what does 'healthy' even mean anymore?

My name is Emily English, a BSc Nutritionist from King's College London and a lover of food. This book is a blend of science, nourishment and, most importantly, joy. I want to inspire you to get into your kitchen and find out how amazing nutrition, balanced eating and delicious food can make you feel without the preconceived ideas of 'healthy'.

Throughout my life, food has always been important to me. Our family of seven would regularly sit and have dinner together around the dining table. If I ever made a recipe, I would always care about how it made others feel. I wanted them to enjoy it, to feel comforted. Food connects us, no matter our age, gender or nationality. It wasn't until my own relationship with food took a blow after a period of working in the fashion industry that I was led to a profound realisation: healthy food should not be about restrictions or labels, it should be about true nourishment for your body and your mind.

That's the philosophy I bring to you in this book. Here, you'll find recipes that break the mould of conventional nutrition dishes. Think vibrant breakfast tacos, sticky halloumi salads and more pasta, less drama. My approach is simple: to create recipes that are a celebration of eating well. Meals that are energising, make you feel 'lighter and brighter' and after a bite you can't help but say that is just SO good.

As you work your way through these recipes, you'll find my favourite dishes inspired by key moments of my life. I want to share with you the joy of cooking, the pleasure of enjoying a meal together and the freedom that comes with a balanced, unrestrictive approach to eating. Let's make meals that bring us happiness, nourish our bodies and feed our souls. Here's to cooking that's not just about filling our plates, but about enriching our lives. Every recipe, every story and every bite in this book is a testament to the simple expression of 'SO GOOD'.

Nutrition Fundamentals

EMBRACING A JOYFUL, SUSTAINABLE APPROACH TO EATING

Let's talk about nutrition and what 'eating well' actually means. Often, these words conjure up thoughts of diets, sacrifices and meals that are anything but fun. But what if I told you it doesn't have to be that way? Eating well can be something you get excited about and enjoy doing for yourself, not something you feel obligated to do.

Through working with countless clients in my career, I've noticed a common thread: everyone is searching for a way of eating that makes them feel good and is sustainable. The problem isn't you, it's the fallacy that dieting is what we need to do when we want to embark on a journey to better health. When it comes to your nutrition, I want you to remember three key things:

1. Start simple and build from there.
2. Tailor it to your life – it should feel like a natural fit.
3. Change doesn't have to be overwhelming. Introduce new habits gradually.

Think of healthy eating as a lifelong journey, not a temporary fix. Yes, it can help us achieve certain goals, like glowing skin or a certain body image, but the heart of it all should be consistency. I often advise you to start by mastering a few recipes that fit into your day-to-day routine. Make them weekly until they feel like second nature, just like brushing your teeth, and these new eating habits and recipes will soon become a natural part of who you are. This is where you will see the biggest change.

My approach isn't about imposing restrictions, it's about cultivating a sense of moderation and mindfulness. When we pause to consider how our food choices will make us feel, we're empowered to make decisions that truly benefit us.

The trap of dietary restriction lies in its tendency to promote an all-or-nothing mindset. If you're too strict and adhering to punishing rules, the desire to 'break free' or 'reward' yourself becomes overwhelming. Remember, nourishing your body with good food is a form of self-care. When you start treating your body with the love and respect it deserves, you'll find balance and joy in healthy eating.

THE FUNDAMENTALS OF HEALTHY EATING

Understand that there is no one-size-fits-all approach to healthy eating. What works for one person might not work for another. As everyone's nutritional needs and responses to foods are unique, take time to think about how certain foods make you feel and adjust your diet accordingly. This could mean tweaking portion sizes, meal timings or the balance of nutrients. Most of us tend to eat three main meals a day with some snacks in between, but there are a few fundamentals that apply to all of us:

- **Focus on a Diverse Diet**
  Incorporate a variety of foods – counting colours, not calories. You will see my recipes are full of variety, which helps support our gut health and, in turn, our mood, our immunity and even our skin. Think about including a range of fruits, vegetables, whole grains, herbs and spices in your cooking. It's about what you can add to your meals, not what you need to take away.

- **Protein and Fibre Focus**
  Start meals with a strong foundation of protein and fibre. Protein and fibre form a dynamic duo in meals, providing the key elements for energy, making us feel fuller for longer, and also benefit our long-term health. Protein is essential not only for building and repairing tissues but also for contributing to satiety. It helps you to feel fuller for longer, reducing the tendency to snack excessively. Beyond its structural roles, protein is crucial in making enzymes and hormones, supporting muscle and bone health, and providing sustained energy. Fibre, which is equally important, is vital for digestive health. It aids in maintaining regular bowel movements and plays a significant role in blood-sugar regulation. High-fibre foods contribute to the feeling of fullness, helping us to manage appetite and also feed our microbiome.

- **Moderation and Not Restriction**
  Avoid the mindset of restriction, as it often leads to an all-or-nothing approach. Healthy eating should include a sense of moderation and enjoyment. It's about nourishing your body and celebrating food, not depriving yourself. There are a few food groups that are associated with negative health effects, such as ultra-processed foods or the overconsumption of refined sugars. Diet context is everything; it's not about eliminating ultra-processed foods, but rather understanding how you can nourish your body predominantly with whole foods while allowing room for less nutritious items in moderation.

In my approach to nutrition and caloric intake, I emphasise the importance of mindful eating over the rigid counting of calories. This perspective encourages focusing on sensible portion sizes and the nutritional content of meals, fostering a healthier relationship with food. By aiming for balanced plates that include a mix of protein, fibre, healthy fats and carbohydrates, we can enjoy a variety of meals that leave us feeling satisfied and energised. In my recipes, I often use vegetable diversity to create dishes that are voluminous and nutritious yet balanced in calories. This approach allows for generous, satisfying portions that are both delicious and healthy.

I encourage listening to your body and paying attention to how food makes you feel, both physically and mentally. By adopting this approach towards nutrition, we learn to make food choices based on nourishment and satisfaction, leading to a more joyful and balanced approach to eating.

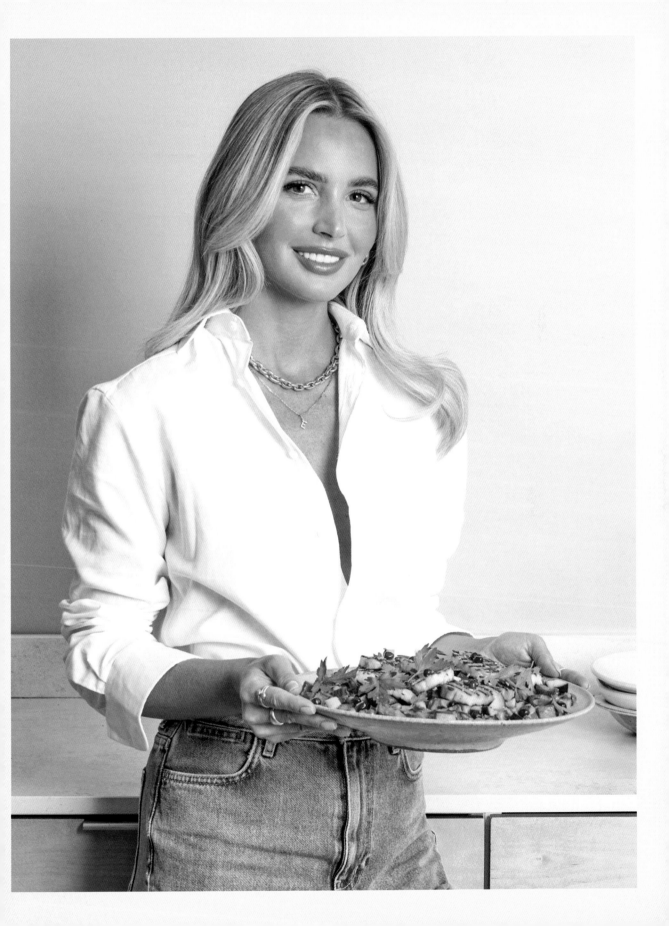

What Could a Day Look Like?

BREAKFAST

- **Start with a strong foundation of protein and fibre:**
  All the recipes in this book have been designed to provide you with the right amount of protein and fibre to keep you full. I love to batch cook my Prepable Breakfast Muffins (see page 36) if I have a busy week ahead, or make a big pot of Matcha Overnight Oats (see page 8) topped with extra fruit and yogurt that will keep me full all morning.

- **Avoid simple carbs:**
  Steer clear of breakfasts that are predominantly simple carbohydrates. Instead of just toast or plain cereal, make my Nutty Granola Clusters (see page 12) paired with thick bio live yogurt and fruit for a sweet but balanced start to your day, or opt for a portion of fluffy Eggy Bread with Tomato Salsa (see page 30).

- **Listen to your hunger cues:**
  If you're not hungry in the morning, don't force yourself to eat a large breakfast. Instead, consider planning a mid-morning snack that is nutritious and satisfying for if you get hungry before lunch. I recommend a slice of the Breakfast Banana Bread Loaf (see page 16) to go.

LUNCH

- **Healthy convenience:**
  Utilise convenient, healthy options like pre-cooked grains, canned legumes and pre-cooked proteins. These can be lifesavers for quick, nutritious lunches. For example, my Sushi Salad (see page 62) uses pre-cooked rice and can be ready in under 15 minutes. I use pre-roasted chicken for my Greek Salad-inspired Chicken Pittas (see page 75) too.

- **Avoid the slump:**
  To combat the sleepy afternoon dip, choose a lunch that balances complex carbohydrates, proteins and healthy fats. I designed the recipes so even the pasta salads are put together in a way that will fuel you but not send you to sleep!

- **Include variety:**
  Avoid the monotony of having the same lunch every day by mixing up ingredients and flavours. There are lots of recipe ideas in this book to inspire you to level up your standard sandwich.

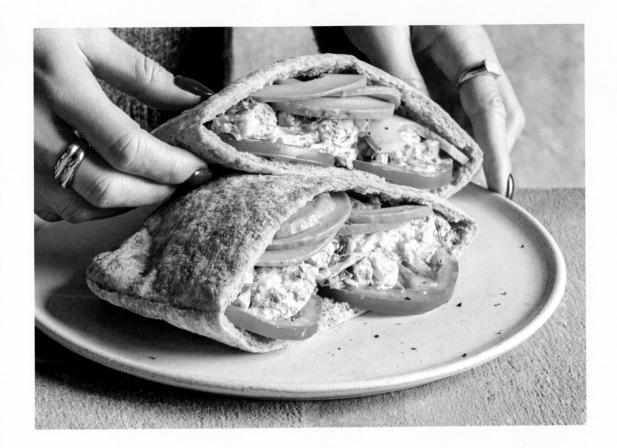

DINNER

- **Plan routine and batch cooking:**
  Establish a routine for dinners that allows for consistency and ease. Batch cooking and using leftovers smartly can save time and reduce stress. For example, my Superfood Vegetarian Bolognese (see page 132) is freezer-friendly, can be paired with pasta or baked into a pie.

- **Vegetable diversity:**
  Focus on including a wide range of colours and types of vegetables, and try to incorporate at least two or three different coloured vegetables into your dinner. This not only makes your plate visually appealing but also ensures a variety of nutrients. My Meatball and Ricotta Al Forno (see page 122) sneaks courgette (zucchini) into the sauce for that vegetable diversity boost.

- **Think about timing and composition:**
  Aim to eat dinner at least two hours before bedtime to aid digestion and sleep. Lean proteins like chicken and fish, or plant-based options like lentils or tofu, can help in the production of serotonin, a precursor to our sleep hormone melatonin. A portion of my Brick Almond Chicken (see page 105) and I'm drifting away in no time!

Understanding Calories and Macronutrients

So what are calories and are they important? Calories are the energy units in the foods we consume, and they play a vital role in maintaining bodily functions. A calorie's impact on our weight and health depends on its source – the macronutrient it comes from – and how the body processes it.

- Protein:
  Typically, about 70–80 per cent of calories from protein are absorbed into the body. For instance, eating 100 calories-worth of chicken provides us with roughly 70 usable calories. This is partly due to the thermic effect of food, where the body uses energy to digest and metabolise protein.

- Carbohydrates:
  The absorption rate of carbohydrates varies around 90–95 per cent, influenced by the fibre content. Fibrous carbs, like whole grains, are absorbed more slowly, providing sustained energy.

- Fats:
  Nearly 100 per cent of the calories from fats are absorbed. While calorie-dense, fats are essential for nutrient absorption and brain health.

FOOD PROCESSING AND CALORIC ABSORPTION

The way food is processed can affect how its calories are absorbed. For example:

- Whole vs. processed foods:
  Consider almonds and almond butter. Whole almonds have a fibrous structure that requires more energy to break them down, leading to fewer net calories being absorbed compared to smoother, more processed almond butter.

- Cooking methods:
  Cooking can also alter calorie availability. For instance, cooked starches are often more easily digestible than raw ones, potentially increasing the calories your body absorbs.

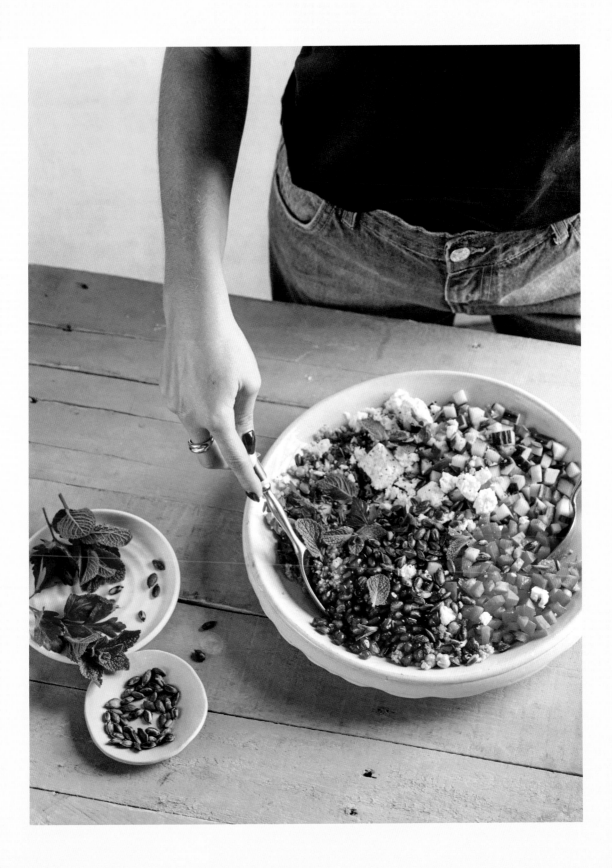

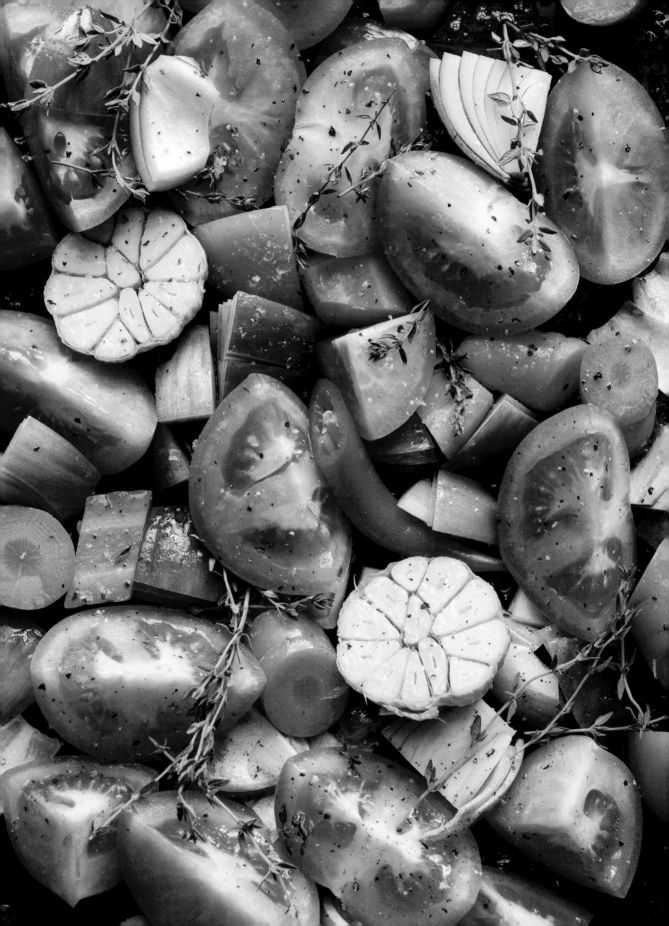

WHY THE GUT IS IMPORTANT

Understanding and nurturing gut health is essential for our overall well-being. Our gut is far more than a digestive centre; it's a complex ecosystem that significantly influences our health, from nutrient absorption and immunity to even our mood and energy levels. The diversity of bacteria in our gut microbiome is a key player in this process, making our dietary choices and lifestyle habits crucial in maintaining gut health.

A varied and plant-rich diet is foundational for a healthy gut. Different types of plant-based foods provide a range of fibres and nutrients, supporting a diverse array of beneficial bacteria. This diversity is vital for a resilient and healthy gut. Incorporating fibre-rich vegetables, fruits, legumes and whole grains in our diet acts as fuel for these good bacteria, enhancing digestion and bolstering our immune system. Fermented foods like yogurt, kefir, sauerkraut and kombucha are also beneficial, introducing helpful bacteria and enzymes that aid digestion and enrich our gut microbiome.

However, gut health isn't solely influenced by what we eat. Lifestyle factors, particularly stress management, play a significant role in maintaining a healthy gut. Chronic stress can upset the balance of gut bacteria, leading to digestive issues, weakened immunity and mood changes. Therefore, incorporating stress-reducing practices, such as mindfulness, ensuring adequate sleep and engaging in regular physical activity, is just as important for gut health.

In summary, nurturing gut health involves a holistic approach:

1. Embrace a diet rich in a variety of plant-based foods and fibres.
2. Include fermented foods to support the gut microbiome.
3. Manage stress through mindful practices, good sleep and regular exercise.

By taking care of our gut health through these measures, we support not just one aspect of our health, but lay a strong foundation for overall physical and mental well-being.

Kitchen Essentials: Tools for Healthier and Easier Cooking

Preparing nutritious and delicious meals is a breeze when you're equipped with the right kitchen tools. Here's a comprehensive guide to essential utensils and appliances, each selected for its practicality and ability to enhance your cooking experience.

EQUIPMENT ESSENTIALS

- **Mixing bowls (various sizes):** A set of mixing bowls is indispensable for everything from combining ingredients to marinating and storing leftovers. Look for bowls with non-slip bases and stackable designs for easy storage.

- **Mini food processor:** Ideal for quickly chopping vegetables and herbs, and making sauces. A mini food processor saves time and is a convenient tool for small-scale preparations.

- **Julienne peeler:** Perfect for creating vegetable noodles or garnishing dishes, a julienne peeler adds a gourmet touch with minimal effort. Choose one with a comfortable grip.

- **Microplane grater:** Essential for finely grating garlic, ginger, citrus zest and hard cheeses, a microplane grater enhances the flavour of your dishes. Get one with a protective cover for safe storage.

- **Oven-safe pans:** Versatile and convenient, oven-safe pans are great for one-pan recipes. Look for nonstick coatings and heat-resistant handles.

- **Air fryer:** For healthier versions of fried foods, an air fryer is a must. It requires minimal oil and offers quick and even cooking.

- **Storage/food containers:** Quality containers are key for meal prep and keeping leftovers fresh, helping to organise your kitchen efficiently. Opt for microwave-safe and BPA-free options.

- **Powerful blender:** A versatile tool for smoothies, soups and more. Choose a blender with multiple speed settings and a durable build.

- **Measuring spoons and cups:** Essential for accurate measurements in cooking and baking. Stainless steel sets are durable and easy to clean.

- **Silicone spatulas:** Heat-resistant and flexible, silicone spatulas ensure you get every last bit from your bowls and pans.

- **Digital scale:** A digital scale is crucial for precision in cooking, especially baking, ensuring you use exact quantities of ingredients.

- **Quality knives:** Invest in a good chef's knife and a paring knife to cover most cutting and chopping needs. Ergonomic handles provide comfort during use.

Equipping your kitchen with these essentials will enhance your culinary experience, making cooking more efficient, enjoyable and conducive to healthy eating. These tools are investments that support your journey in creating wholesome and satisfying meals.

PANTRY ESSENTIALS

- **Extra virgin olive oil:** I always opt for a bottle of high-quality extra virgin olive oil, which I find myself using every day for dressings and cooking. The trick is to choose oil in dark, non-glass bottles to maintain its quality. You should look for bitter tasting notes as a sign of high antioxidant and polyphenol content. A drizzle of olive oil can elevate a simple salad or add the finishing touch to a warm soup; a 3g portion boosts the absorption of fat-soluble vitamins A, D, E and K.

- **Canned legumes:** No pantry is complete without a selection of canned legumes. Beans, chickpeas and lentils are not only quick protein fixes but also pack a punch with fibre, iron and essential minerals. They're perfect for throwing together a last-minute chilli or enhancing a salad for a protein-rich meal.

- **Whole grains:** Staples like quinoa, brown rice and wholegrain pastas aren't just versatile, they're full of health benefits. Rich in dietary fibre, they aid digestion and promote satiety – but are also packed with nutrients like B vitamins and magnesium. I include them in meals for their nutritional value and ability to stabilise blood sugar, which is beneficial for energy levels.

- **Core flavour items:** My kitchen is never without flavour boosters like miso, soy sauce and a variety of herbs and spices. Miso adds a depth of flavour to soups and marinades, while soy sauce is my go-to for an Asian twist. Herbs and spices are the backbone of cooking, offering both health benefits and incredible flavours. As you work your way through the recipes in this book, you'll see a lot of my core flavour items are used across multiple meals.

- **My three hero items are capers, olives and sun-dried tomatoes.** Capers add a tangy zing to sauces and salads, plus they're packed with antioxidants. Olives, a key ingredient in Mediterranean cooking, are rich in heart-healthy fats and vitamin E. Sun-dried tomatoes transform pastas and salads while providing vitamins C and K, iron and antioxidants. These little additions are my secret to adding a special flavour boost, as well as providing extra nutrition.

- **Nuts and seeds:** Nuts and seeds are little nuggets of nutrition. Almonds, walnuts, chia and flaxseeds (linseeds) are excellent for a fibre boost. I sprinkle them on oatmeal, blend them into smoothies or simply snack on them for a quick energy boost. Their healthy fats, proteins and essential nutrients make them an invaluable part of my diet and an easy way to boost diversity.

- **Oats:** I use oats a lot, from breakfast to baking. It's always worth having a bag of oats in your cupboard. I prefer jumbo oats for their satiety, slower digestion and lower impact on blood sugar levels. They contain something called beta-glucans, a type of soluble fibre that's excellent for heart health and lowering cholesterol. Blend into flour to use in many of my breakfast loaves and muffins.

- **Frozen fruits and vegetables:** The misconception that frozen fruits and vegetables are inferior to fresh ones couldn't be further from the truth. Freezing actually locks in all the nutrients. Some of my go-to freezer items include berries, green peas, green beans, grilled Mediterranean vegetables, sweetcorn and spinach. They are not only convenient for adding to smoothies, but I often use them for sauces, ragùs and curries.

- **Long-lasting proteins**: In my kitchen, you'll find long-lasting proteins to bulk out my meals, including things like canned tuna, frozen prawns and tofu. Canned tuna is great for quick sandwiches or salads, while frozen prawns can be thrown into curries and pasta sauces. Tofu, a versatile plant-based protein, is excellent in stir-fry recipes or grilled, and keeps for around 2 months in your refrigerator. Protein is key in our meals to keep us full and sustained for longer.

- **Thick natural yogurt**: Thick, creamy natural yogurt is a staple in my refrigerator. It's not only perfect for breakfast bowls but also versatile enough for dressings and baking. Packed with protein, calcium and probiotics, it's a nutritious addition to many meals that I use a lot. My preference is bio live for extra gut health benefits.

- **Whole grains:** Quinoa, brown rice and wholegrain pasta are my go-to grains. They are not just the foundation of a hearty meal but also come packed with fibre, B vitamins and essential minerals for sustained energy throughout the day. They will sit forever in your pantry and I often like to batch cook them on a Sunday night to pair with meals throughout the week.

- **Vinegar:** Be it apple cider, balsamic or red wine, vinegar is not only essential for brightening up dressings and marinades, but it also comes with notable health benefits. Apple cider vinegar, for instance, is noted for its potential in aiding digestion and regulating blood sugar levels. I use vinegar to make my own pickles, as some store-bought ones can be quite high in salt and sugar. Pickles can aid satiety and help to control blood sugar spikes. Plus, if you opt for fermented pickles, there are additional benefits for our gut health.

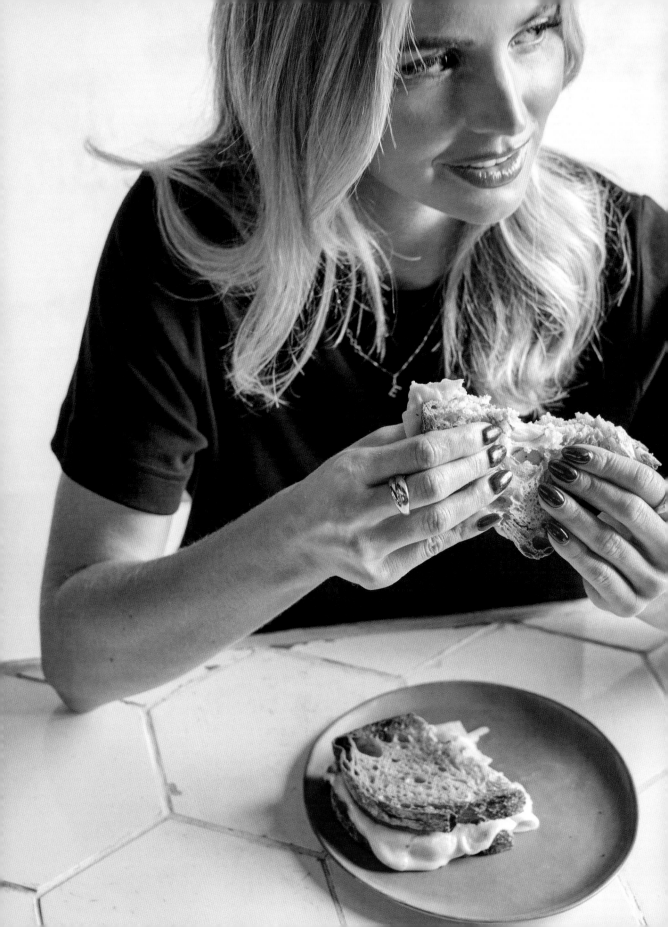

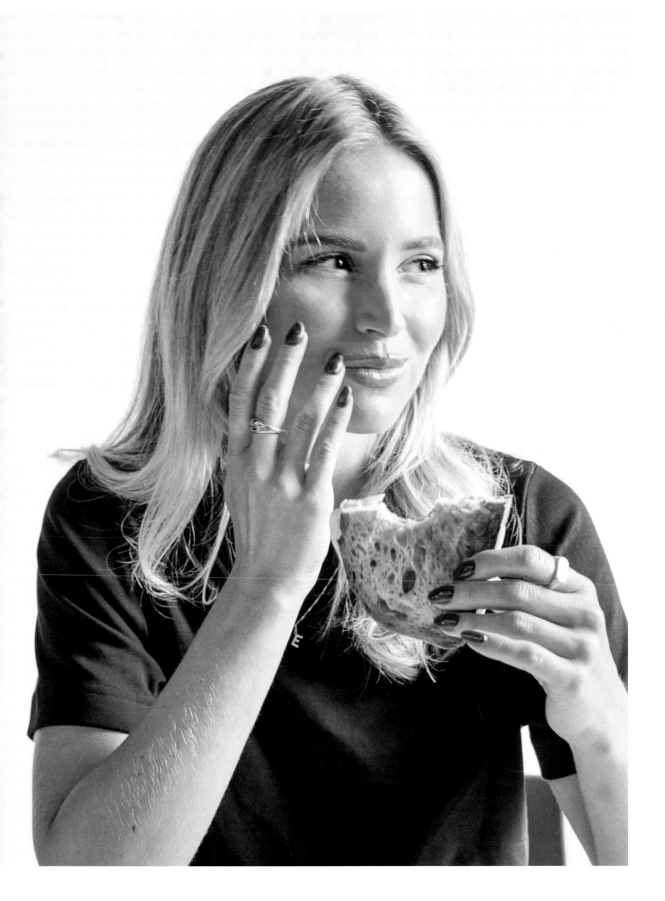

02-39

Breakfast

02   Fluffy Ricotta Lemon Pancakes

04   Tomato and Ricotta Breakfast Bowls

07   Blueberry Crumble Breakfast Oat Bars

08   Matcha Overnight Oats

09   Chia Berry Compote

11   Gut Food Smoothie Bowl

12   Nutty Granola Clusters

15   Chocolate Orange Oats with Citrus Honey

16   Breakfast Banana Bread Loaf

18   Chopped Egg Breakfast Toast

21   Tray-bake English Breakfast

22   Lighter Sausage Breakfast Bagels

25   Smoked Salmon and Cream Cheese Omelette

26   Pan con Tomate

29   Sun-dried Tomato Shakshuka

30   Eggy Bread with Tomato Salsa

32   Hot Honey Halloumi Avocado Toast

35   Morning Tacos

36   Prepable Breakfast Muffins

38   Crispy Feta Eggs

Fluffy Ricotta Lemon Pancakes

Serves 4

Time:
25 minutes

Macros:
Under 250kcal,
12g protein per serving
(2 pancakes per
serving)

These are the best pancakes I have ever eaten. Melt-in-your-mouth soft, so light, and seriously addictive while staying balanced. Pair with fresh fruits or my Chia Berry Compote (see page 9). Top with a drizzle of syrup or honey. These can also be made in advance and heated up for ease – simply microwave or flash in a hot pan.

250g (generous 1 cup) ricotta cheese

125ml (½ cup) semi-skimmed milk

2 large free-range eggs, separated

100g (¾ cup) plain (all-purpose) flour

1 teaspoon baking powder

Zest of 1 unwaxed lemon

Pinch of salt

Olive oil, for cooking

To serve

4 tablespoons Chia Berry Compote (see page 9)

Drizzle of maple syrup or honey

- Separate out 75g (⅓ cup) of ricotta and set to one side. In a large mixing bowl, beat the remaining ricotta, the milk and egg yolks to form a smooth batter. Gently mix in the dry ingredients (flour, baking powder, lemon zest and a pinch of salt).

- In a separate, clean bowl, whisk the egg whites until soft, white and fluffy (around 2 minutes), then fold them into the batter. Using a teaspoon, dollop little blobs of the reserved ricotta into the bowl and fold through 5 or 6 times, trying not to break the ricotta up. We want little surprise pockets when eating the pancakes.

- Place a nonstick frying pan over a medium heat and brush with a little olive oil. Dollop a large scoop of batter into the pan. Cook for around 2 minutes on each side until golden and risen. If your pan is big enough, you can cook multiple pancakes at once.

- To serve, spoon over 1 tablespoon of chia berry compote and drizzle over some maple syrup or honey.

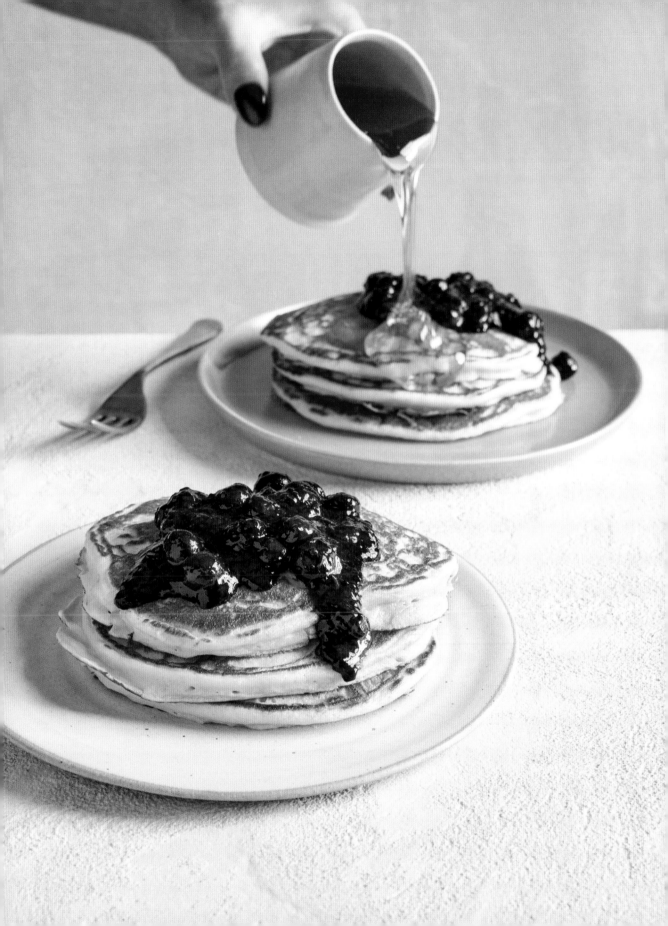

Tomato and Ricotta Breakfast Bowls

Serves 2

Time:
20 minutes

Macros:
Under 360kcal,
26g protein per serving

Bright and fresh cherry tomatoes paired with creamy ricotta with fried eggs. Break the yolks into the ricotta and scoop up with a slice of toast. Ricotta provides calcium and protein, while tomatoes are packed with antioxidants. It's a perfect combination that both fuels and satisfies, leaving you set for the morning.

6 tablespoons ricotta cheese

Zest and juice of ½ unwaxed lemon

30g (1oz) Parmesan cheese, grated, plus extra to finish

2 teaspoons olive oil

1 garlic clove, unpeeled

2 large handfuls of cherry tomatoes, cut in half

2 tablespoons balsamic vinegar

Large handful of basil leaves, chopped

4 medium free-range eggs

2 slices of bread of choice

Salt and pepper

- In a bowl, mix the ricotta cheese with the lemon zest and juice and Parmesan and season to taste with salt and pepper.

- Heat the olive oil in a frying pan over a medium heat, and add the unpeeled garlic clove. Throw in the cherry tomatoes and sauté for 5 minutes, adding the balsamic vinegar and sautéing for another 5 minutes, tossing from time to time until they soften. Finish with a small handful of chopped basil to wilt. Remove the tomatoes and wilted basil, discard the garlic and set to one side to keep warm. In the same pan, fry the eggs.

- Toast the bread.

- To serve, spoon the ricotta mix onto a plate, add the fried eggs, then the blistered tomatoes and basil, and finish with a little flurry of Parmesan and extra freshly ground pepper. Serve using the toast to mop up all the lovely lemony ricotta.

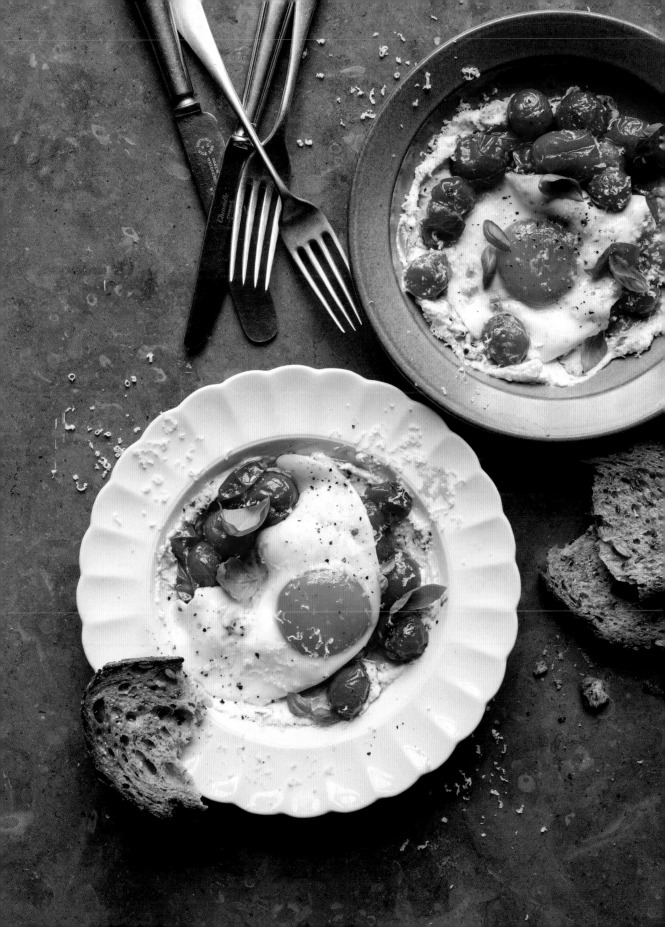

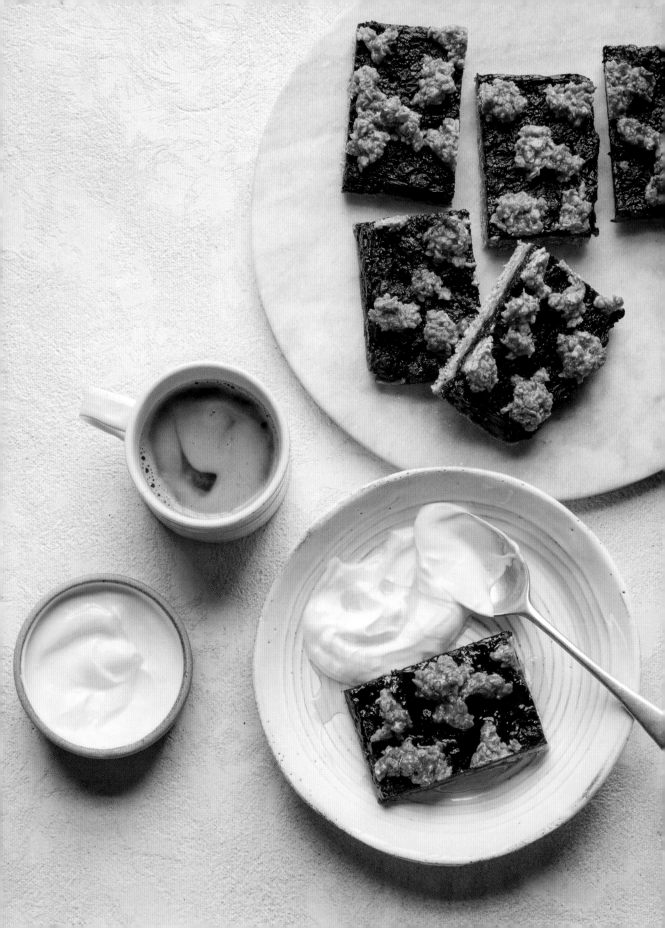

Blueberry Crumble Breakfast Oat Bars

When it comes to sweet breakfast ideas, these oat bars are one of my favourites. Essentially all the ingredients you put in your porridge with a layer of sticky blueberry compote. Serve with a big dollop of natural yogurt for filling protein and you have the perfect breakfast.

Makes 4

Time:
35 minutes

Macros:
Under 350kcal,
10g protein per bar

400g (14oz) frozen blueberries

1 heaped tablespoon chia seeds

2 teaspoons vanilla extract

1 large ripe banana (if not ripe add more sugar to taste)

3 tablespoons smooth peanut butter

½ teaspoon baking powder

2–3 tablespoons fine sugar, honey or sweetener (I like erythritol)

Pinch of salt

4 tablespoons semi-skimmed milk

130g (1⅓ cups) rolled oats (not instant oats!)

30g (4 tablespoons) plain (all-purpose) or oat flour

1 teaspoon ground cinnamon

To serve

Thick natural yogurt (0% fat or full fat)

Drizzle of maple syrup or honey

- Start by gently simmering the blueberries in a pan. Once defrosted and bubbling, stir in the chia seeds and 1 teaspoon vanilla extract. Allow the mixture to cool.

- Preheat the oven to 190°C/170°C fan (375°F) Gas Mark 5 (unless using an air fryer). Line a baking tin, about 20 x 20cm (8 x 8 inches), with nonstick baking paper.

- For the oat layer, mash the banana in a bowl using a fork until smooth. Add the remaining vanilla extract, the peanut butter, baking powder, sugar, salt and milk and stir to create your wet mixture. In another bowl, merge the oats, flour and cinnamon. Gently incorporate the wet mixture into the dry ingredients, ensuring you get a cohesive, slightly sticky batter.

- Transfer this batter to the lined baking tin, reserving about a third, and spread evenly. Spread the cooled blueberry mixture over the top.

- Using your hands, form little clusters with the reserved batter and scatter them on top of the blueberry layer.

- Bake in the oven for 15–20 minutes until you achieve a golden hue. Alternatively, cook at 150°C (300°F) in an air fryer for about 15 minutes.

- Once done, allow to cool in the tin. Cut into 4 even squares or 6 rectangles, and serve with protein-rich thick natural yogurt and a light drizzle of maple syrup or honey. These bars can be stored in an airtight container in the refrigerator and enjoyed for up to 4 days.

Matcha Overnight Oats

Serves 1

Time:
5 minutes, plus
overnight chilling

Macros:
Under 300kcal,
19g protein

These vibrant green oats are a wonderful way to incorporate matcha into your mornings. I love matcha for its powerful antioxidant hit, nutrient density and slow-release caffeine. This is a quick-to-prepare and easy breakfast solution for busy mornings. Batch make and keep in the refrigerator for 2 days.

35g (⅓ cup) jumbo oats

100ml (scant ½ cup) milk of choice

100g (½ cup) thick natural yogurt, plus extra if needed

½ teaspoon matcha powder

Handful of raspberries or blueberries, plus extra to serve

1 teaspoon whole flaxseeds (linseeds)

½ teaspoon ground cinnamon

1 teaspoon chia seeds

1 teaspoon honey or sweetener of choice

Optional

Add a scoop of protein powder to make this even more filling

- Mix all the ingredients in a bowl.

- Cover and store in the refrigerator overnight.

- In the morning, adjust the consistency with more yogurt, if needed.

- Add extra berries on top and serve.

Chia Berry Compote

Serves 6

Time:
10 minutes

Macros:
Under 50kcal
per serving

I love to prep this compote every week as it makes the ideal topper for oats, natural yogurt and even on toast. It is a great sweet, but lower sugar, option packed full of fibre, vitamins and lots of antioxidants. This is a staple recipe for me and uses the convenience of frozen fruit too. Feel free to get creative and try different fruits and spices.

400g (14oz) frozen blueberries or raspberries

1 heaped tablespoon chia seeds

1 teaspoon vanilla extract

- Tip the frozen berries into a pan and gently heat, allowing them to defrost. Once defrosted, bring to a gentle simmer.

- Stir in the chia seeds and vanilla, and let it simmer for a few more minutes. Remove from the heat and let the mix cool to thicken.

- Transfer to a sealable jar and store for up to 1 week in the refrigerator.

Note:
This Chia Berry Compote is amazing with pancakes (see page 2), granola (see page 12), natural yogurt and more!

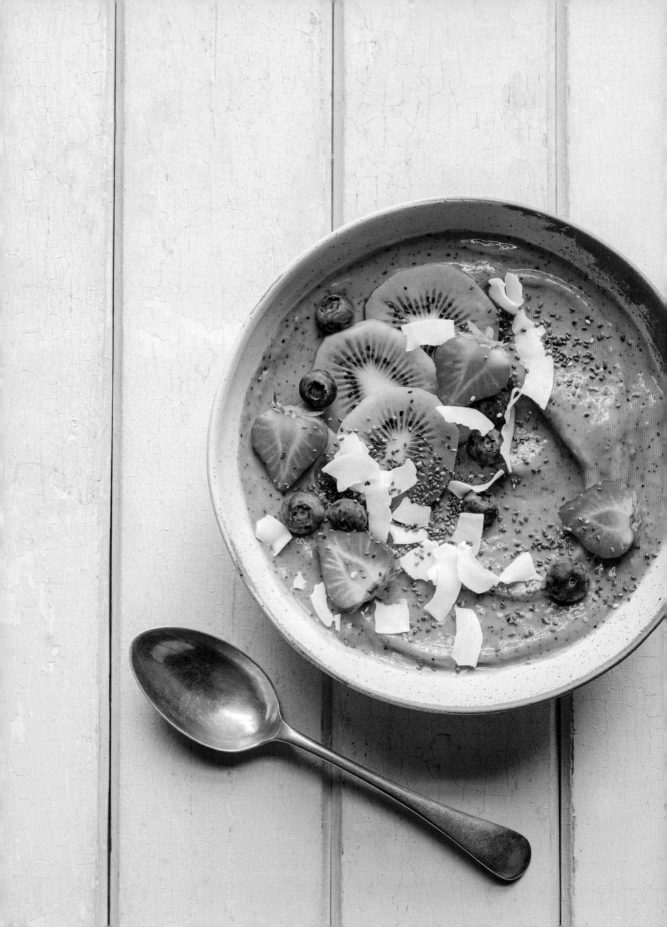

Gut Food
Smoothie Bowl

This smoothie bowl is so bright and refreshing, packed with fibre-rich raspberries and blueberries and high-protein natural yogurt, with the freedom to top with whatever you like. I love to add fresh fruits, a swirl of nut butter and a sprinkle of crunchy seeds or nuts. Not only does this bowl look beautiful, but it's also a powerhouse of nutrients and fuel for the gut. To boost the protein, simply add a scoop of protein powder into the base before blending.

Serves 1

Time:
10 minutes

Macros:
Under 250kcal,
13g protein for the
smoothie base

100g (3½oz) frozen raspberries

50g (1¾oz) frozen blueberries

50g (1¾oz) frozen mango

½ ripe banana

100g (½ cup) strained natural yogurt (0% fat) or skyr

For the optional toppings

Sliced fresh fruit of choice

1 teaspoon nut butter of choice

1 teaspoon seeds of choice

1 tablespoon coconut flakes

- Add the frozen fruit and banana, then the yogurt, to a blender. Blend and pulse, pushing the fruit down and mixing if it gets stuck. Be patient as it will all blend together eventually. Avoid adding extra liquid as this will prevent you from having a thick smoothie bowl.

- Spoon the smoothie into a bowl and add your favourite toppings.

Nutty Granola Clusters

Makes 20
portions

Time:
30 minutes

Macros:
Under 160kcal,
5g protein per serving

Struggling to find a low-sugar, protein-rich granola off the shelves? Try my easy-to-make Nutty Granola Clusters, packed with protein and gut-loving fibre. The secret to these divine, crunchy clusters is actually egg whites. Pair this granola with my Chia Berry Compote (see page 9) and thick natural yogurt for a delicious, nourishing breakfast. Store in an airtight jar for up to 1 month.

200g (2 cups) jumbo oats

100g (¾ cup) mixed seeds (pumpkin, sunflower, etc.)

150g (1¼ cups) mixed skin-on whole hazelnuts and cashew nuts

100g (scant ½ cup) smooth peanut butter

2 medium free-range egg whites

100g (⅓ cup) honey

10 drops of liquid stevia

1 tablespoon ground cinnamon (optional)

To serve

Thick natural yogurt (0% fat or full fat)

Chia Berry Compote (see page 9, using frozen summer fruits)

- Combine all the dry and wet ingredients in a bowl until everything is thoroughly coated.

- For the air fryer method: Lay a sheet of nonstick baking paper in the air fryer. Use your hands to evenly distribute the granola mixture in a single layer on the baking paper, ensuring some clusters remain. Avoid overcrowding. Air-fry in batches at 120°C (250°F) for 12–17 minutes, stirring occasionally, until golden and crisp. Granola will become crisper as it cools but should retain a bit of chew. Allow to cool before storing in an airtight container for up to 1 month.

- For the oven method: Preheat the oven to 150°C/130°C fan (300°F) Gas Mark 2. Spread the granola on a baking tray lined with nonstick baking paper. Bake in the oven for 15–25 minutes, stirring occasionally, until golden and crisp. Allow to cool before storing in an airtight container for up to 1 month.

- Serve the granola over thick natural yogurt and top with a spoonful of compote or however you like.

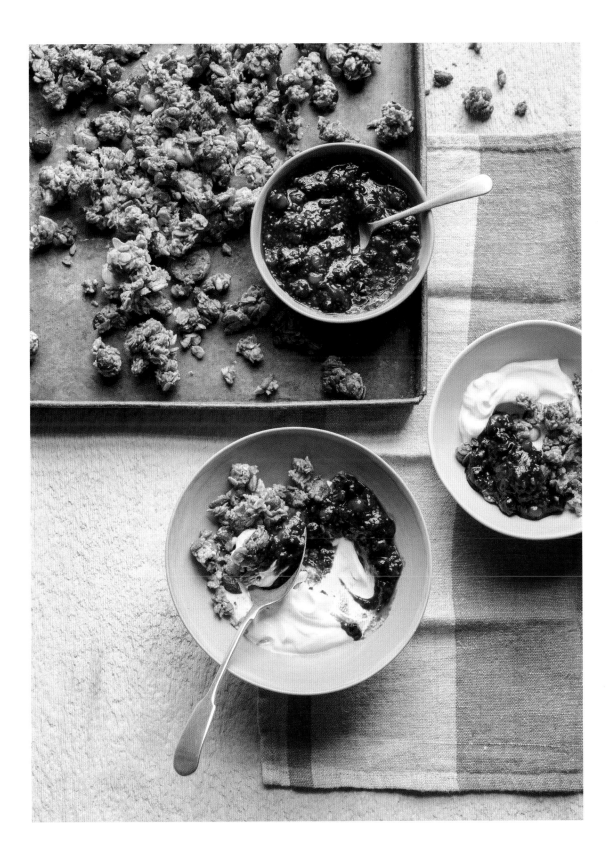

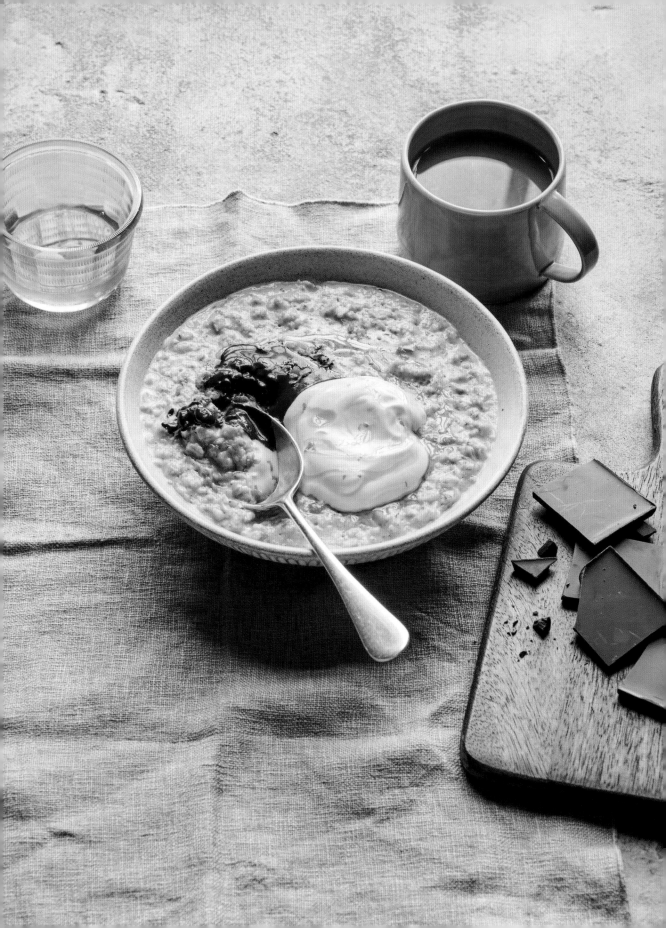

Chocolate Orange Oats with Citrus Honey

Elevate your breakfast oats with these vitamin C-rich, orange-spiced oats. The comforting combination of cinnamon, orange zest, dark chocolate and honey is just so perfect for breakfast, topped with a dollop of natural yogurt and an extra grating of orange zest. Did you know that dark chocolate contains high levels of polyphenols which help support a healthy gut?

Serves 1

Time:
10 minutes

Macros:
Under 350kcal,
15g protein

35g (⅓ cup) jumbo oats

1 tablespoon ground cinnamon

Zest and juice of 1 orange

150ml (⅔ cup) semi-skimmed milk or milk of choice

1 heaped teaspoon honey

1 square of dark chocolate (70% cocoa content)

1 tablespoon thick natural yogurt

Optional

Increase the protein content by adding a scoop of your favourite protein powder

- In a saucepan, combine the oats, cinnamon and orange zest.

- Add in the juice from half the orange along with the milk, and bring to a gentle simmer.

- Cook until the oats have softened and reached a porridge-like consistency, around 2–3 minutes.

- In a separate bowl, mix the honey with the remaining orange juice.

- Transfer the cooked porridge to a serving bowl.

- Top with the square of dark chocolate, followed by a drizzle of the orange-honey mixture, then finish with a dollop of yogurt.

Breakfast Banana Bread Loaf

One of my most popular prepable and transportable recipes, my Breakfast Banana Bread Loaf is full of blood sugar-balancing oats, walnuts and olive oil for a nutritionally complete breakfast. It pairs perfectly with a dollop of natural yogurt and a drizzle of nut butter and will keep in an airtight container for over a week. Cake for breakfast anyone?

Makes 10 slices/ portions

Time:
55 minutes, plus resting

Macros:
Under 250kcal, 4g protein per slice

---

3 large overripe bananas, plus 1 extra banana to finish

5 tablespoons olive oil, plus extra for greasing

80g (¼ cup) honey

150g (1½ cups) rolled oats

75g (generous ½ cup) plain (all-purpose) flour

1 heaped teaspoon baking powder

½ teaspoon bicarbonate of soda (baking soda)

40g (⅓ cup) walnuts, roughly chopped

2 tablespoons pumpkin seeds

• Preheat the oven to 200°C/180°C fan (400°F) Gas Mark 6. Lightly grease a 900g (2lb) nonstick loaf tin (pan).

• In a bowl, use a fork to prepare a wet mixture with 3 mashed bananas, the olive oil and honey until evenly combined.

• In a separate bowl, blend the oats into a flour-like consistency, then add the rest of the dry ingredients, including the nuts and seeds.

• Gently fold the wet mix into the dry ingredients until just combined, taking care not to over-mix.

• Allow the mixture to rest for about 5 minutes, then pour it into the greased loaf tin. Slice the remaining banana in half lengthways and place on top of the cake.

• Bake in the oven for 20 minutes, then loosely cover with foil and bake for an additional 20 minutes, or until a skewer inserted into the centre of the loaf comes out clean. Allow the loaf to rest in the tin for 30 minutes.

• Turn the loaf out of the tin. Cut into slices and serve your warm Breakfast Banana Bread Loaf with natural yogurt, nut butter and frozen raspberries for an extra burst of flavour.

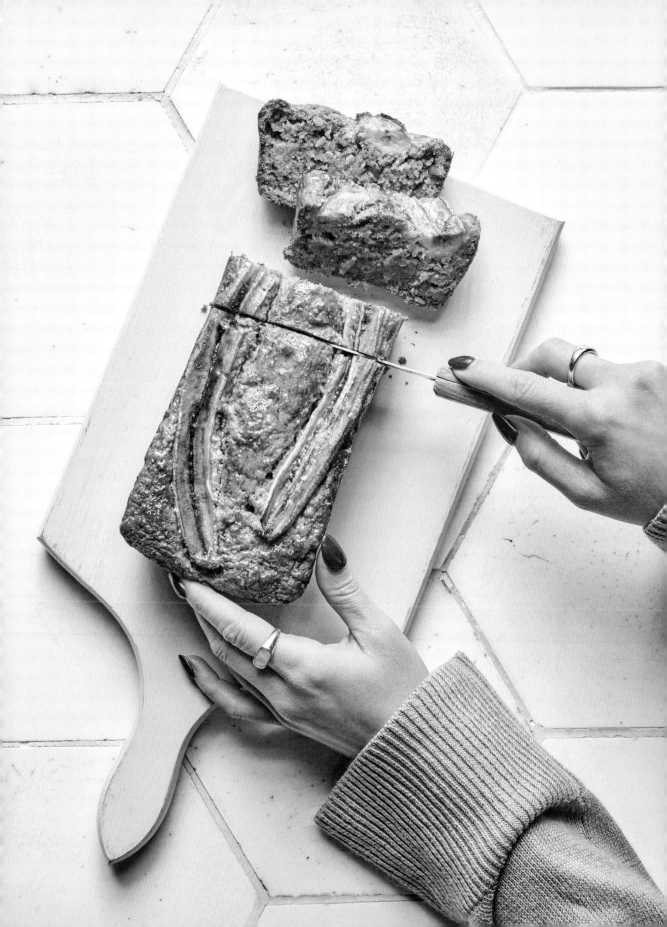

Chopped Egg Breakfast Toast

Serves 1

Time:
15 minutes

Macros:
Under 250kcal,
17g protein

Perfect for breakfast and quick to assemble, my chopped egg mix is a satisfying combination of creamy yogurt, fresh tomatoes with a slight kick from dried chilli flakes and the fresh touch of basil. High in protein and nutrient dense. You can actually prep this filling and store it in the refrigerator for up to 3 days for quick breakfasts throughout the week.

2 large free-range eggs

Handful of cherry tomatoes, finely diced

1 tablespoon thick natural yogurt (0% fat or full fat)

Juice of ½ lemon

1 small spring onion (scallion), finely diced

A few sprigs of basil, leaves finely chopped

2 crispbreads or a toasted slice of bread of choice

Salt and pepper

Pinch of dried red chilli flakes, to finish

- Place the eggs in a small pan and cover with cold water. Bring to the boil, then reduce the heat and let them simmer for 8 minutes for a slightly soft centre. Once boiled, transfer to a bowl of cold water to cool, then peel them and roughly chop.

- In a mixing bowl, combine the roughly chopped eggs, diced cherry tomatoes and the yogurt. Season with a generous pinch of salt and pepper, then squeeze in a little lemon juice and fold in the spring onion and basil. Mix gently, ensuring the ingredients meld together but retain the chunkiness of the eggs and tomatoes.

- Lay out your crispbreads or toasted slice of bread. Generously heap the egg and tomato mixture on top.

- Finish with a sprinkle of chilli flakes for extra heat.

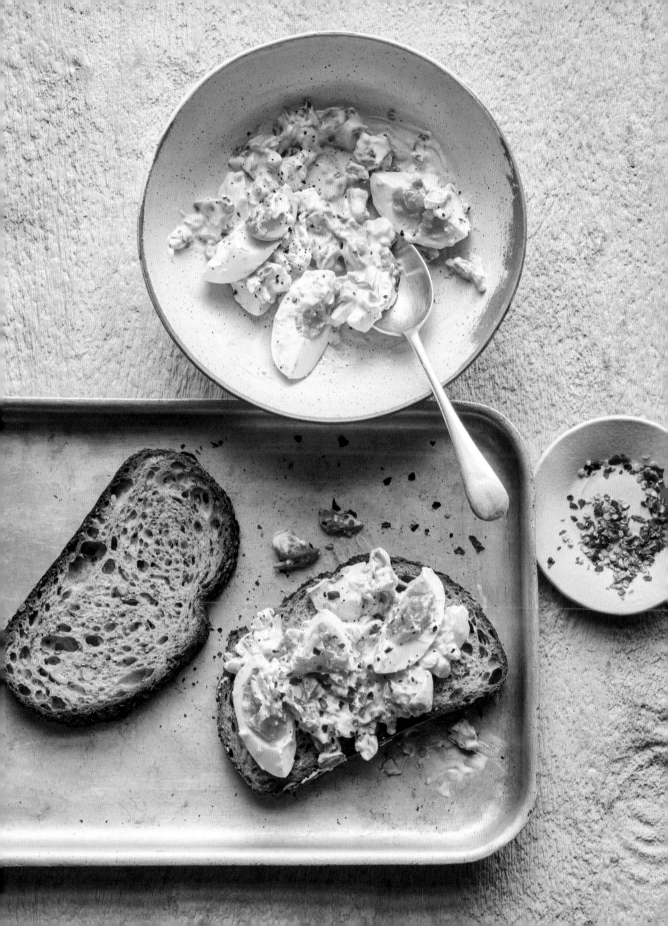

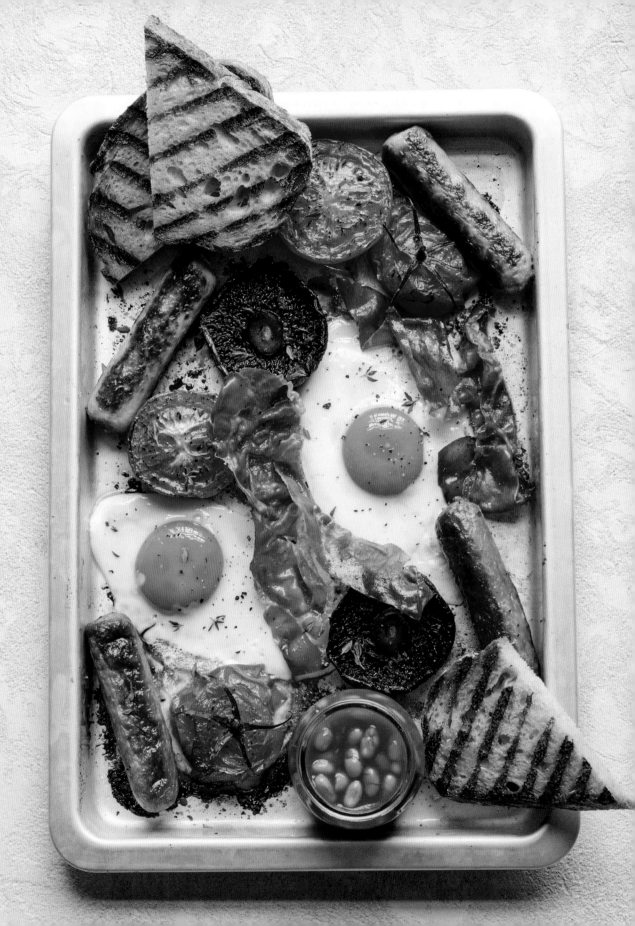

Tray-bake
English Breakfast

Serves 2

Time:
25 minutes

Macros:
Under 450kcal,
30g protein per serving

Transform the traditional English breakfast with this lightened-up tray-baked version. It's perfect for lazy weekend brunches – simply throw everything into the oven until golden and the eggs are oozing, plus there is always the option to pair with some baked beans.

1 tablespoon balsamic vinegar

¼ teaspoon garlic granules

1 teaspoon honey

2 sprigs of thyme, leaves stripped

2 large portobello mushrooms

2 large tomatoes, halved

1 teaspoon dried oregano

2 lighter pork sausages or 4 chicken chipolata-style sausages

2 slices of Parma ham, torn

Good olive oil, for drizzling

2 medium free-range eggs

2 slices of bread of choice

Salt and pepper

- Preheat the oven to 220°C/200°C fan (425°F) Gas Mark 7.

- In a bowl, combine the balsamic vinegar, garlic granules, honey and thyme. Stir well.

- Coat the mushrooms thoroughly in the mixture.

- Grab a large nonstick baking tray or ovenproof dish. Add the halved tomatoes, cut-side up, and sprinkle with the oregano, then place the mushrooms around the tomatoes, and arrange the sausages and Parma ham ribbons in a single layer. Drizzle everything with olive oil and season with salt and pepper.

- Bake in the oven for 15–20 minutes or until everything is looking golden, turning the sausages halfway through for even colouring.

- Make 2 small spaces in the tray/dish and crack an egg into each. Bake for an additional 5–8 minutes or until the egg whites are set. Meanwhile, toast the bread.

- Remove from the oven and serve with the toast and your favourite condiments. Baked beans optional!

Lighter Sausage Breakfast Bagels

Serves 4

Time:
25 minutes

Macros:
Under 450 kcal,
24g protein per bagel

Enhance your breakfast routine with these Lighter Sausage Breakfast Bagels. Packed with protein and essential nutrients, these bagels are a healthier twist on a classic favourite. The sausage offers a hearty dose of protein, there is vitamin C from the tomatoes and spinach, while the bagel provides energy-fuelling complex carbohydrates. When paired together, you get a meal that satisfies your morning hunger and also nourishes your body for the day ahead.

10 chicken chipolata-style sausages
1–2 large ripe tomatoes, sliced
4 wholegrain bagels, sliced horizontally in half
4 slices of Cheddar cheese
100g (3½oz) baby spinach leaves
Salt and pepper

- Skin the sausages and shape the sausagemeat into 4 patties that will fit the size of your bagels.

- Season the tomato slices with a touch of salt and rest them on kitchen paper to absorb the excess moisture.

- Gently toast the bagels. While still warm, take the base of each bagel and lay a slice of cheese on top.

- In a frying pan over a medium heat, sear the patties for 3–4 minutes on each side until they're golden and fully cooked through. Place them over the cheese slices. In the same pan, briefly sauté the spinach just until it wilts.

- Finish by placing a few tomato slices and a portion of the wilted spinach on top of each patty, then replace the bagel lids. Eat immediately or cool, then seal and wrap in foil. Store refrigerated for up to 3 days, or freeze for future enjoyment for up to 3 months. Make sure to fully defrost and reheat your leftovers, ensuring food is piping hot all the way through.

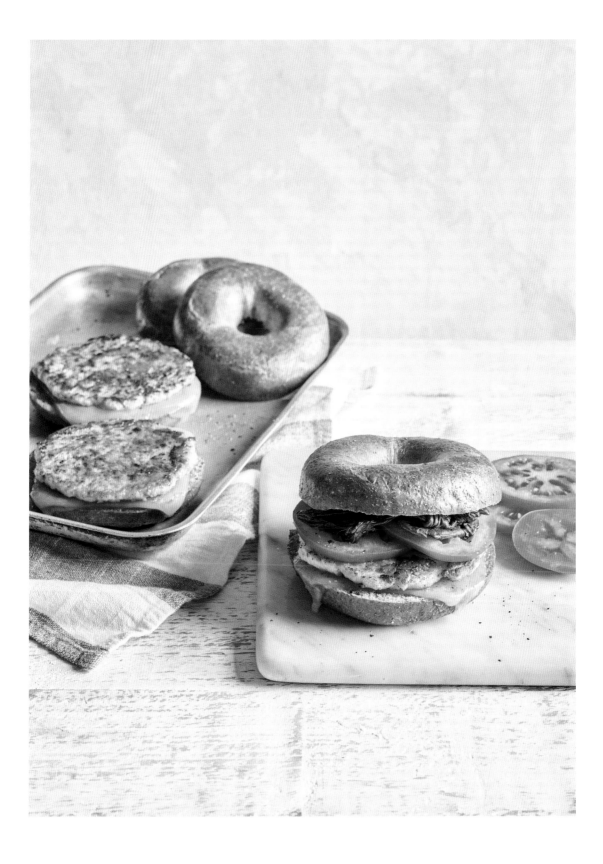

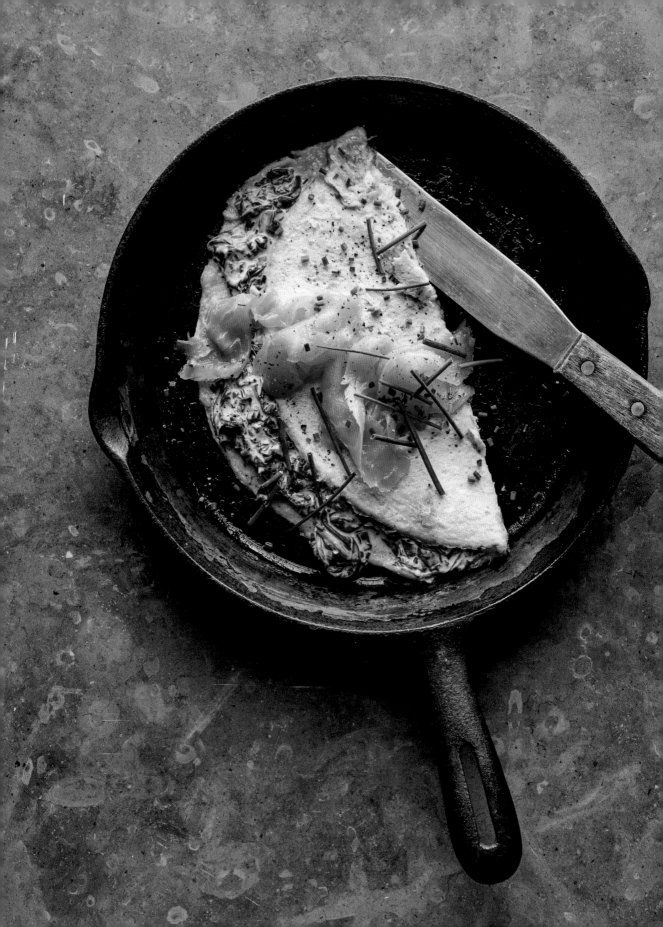

Smoked Salmon and Cream Cheese Omelette

Serves 1

Time:
10 minutes

Macros:
Under 300kcal,
26g protein

This omelette is both nourishing and filling – a creamy blend of spinach, garlic-spiked cream cheese and omega-3-rich smoked salmon all folded into an omelette. Ready in under 10 minutes, it's a quick and simple breakfast perfect for busy but delicious mornings.

Ingredients
2 medium free-range eggs
Large handful of baby spinach leaves
1 heaped tablespoon garlic and herb cream cheese (either low-fat or regular)
1 teaspoon finely chopped chives
50g (1¾oz) smoked salmon, cut into strips
Salt and pepper

- In a bowl, whisk the eggs with a fork and season with salt and pepper, then set aside.

- Sauté the spinach with a pinch of salt in a nonstick frying pan over a medium heat until wilted. Remove from the pan and place into a separate bowl.

- Mix the cooked spinach with the cream cheese and chives.

- Pour the whisked eggs into the hot frying pan and allow to set for 2 minutes, then spoon over the spinach mixture and top with the smoked salmon.

- Fold the omelette in half to close, and allow to cook for a final minute before serving.

Pan con Tomate

My Pan con Tomate is my quick escape to Spain without leaving the kitchen. A toasted slice of my favourite bread rubbed with garlic, then topped with antioxidant-rich tomato pulp. Throw on some protein-packed soft-boiled eggs, a drizzle of heart-healthy olive oil, and a sprinkle of chives. Not only is it delicious, but it's also a nutritious kick-start to any day. Simple, yet so good!

Serves 1

Time:
15 minutes

Macros:
Under 300kcal,
16g protein

---

1 medium-sized tomato, at room temperature

2 medium free-range eggs

1 slice of bread of choice

½ garlic clove

1 teaspoon extra virgin olive oil

A few chives, snipped

Flaky sea salt

- Cut the tomato in half. Using the large side of a box grater, grate the tomato (flesh side against the grater) and collect the pulp in a sieve (strainer). Discard the skin. Season the pulp with flaky salt and allow it to drain while you prepare the eggs.

- Bring a small pan of water to the boil. Gently add the eggs and let them simmer for 6 minutes. Immediately transfer them to cold water to cool, then peel.

- Toast the bread. While it's still warm, lightly rub one side with the cut side of the half garlic clove.

- Mix the strained tomato pulp with the olive oil and top the toasted bread with the tomato pulp, seasoning again with a pinch of salt.

- Place the eggs on top, cut them in half, then sprinkle with snipped chives.

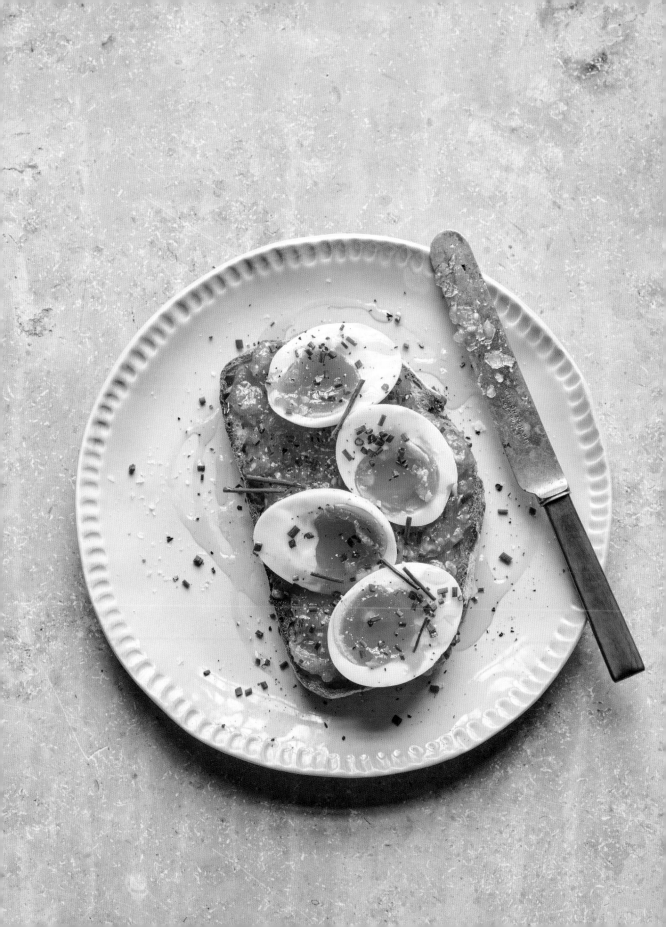

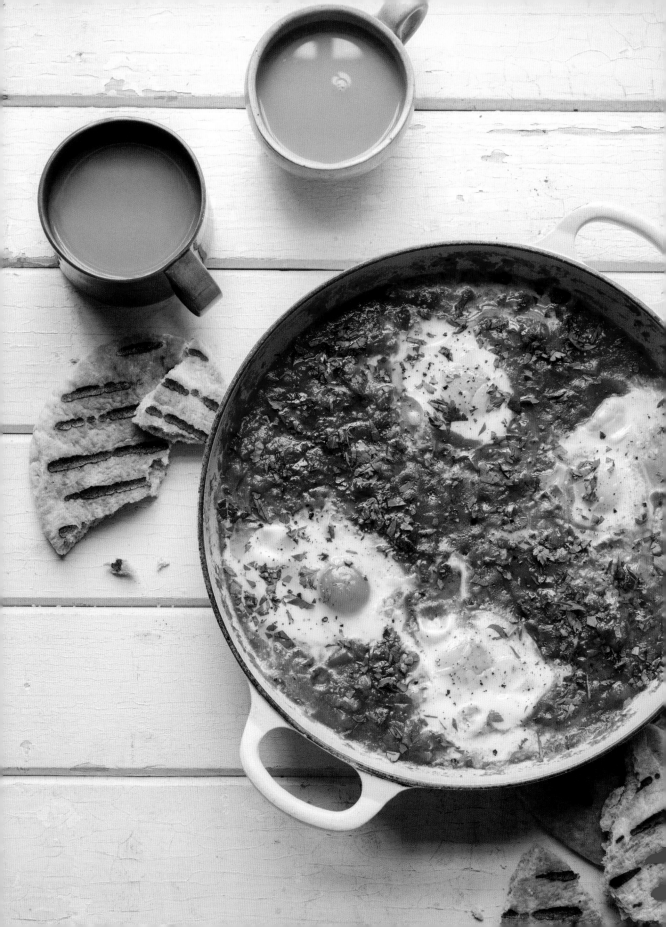

Sun-dried Tomato Shakshuka

Serves 4

Time:
30 minutes

Macros:
Under 350kcal,
10g protein per serving

This is one of those recipes that just belongs in the centre of the table on a Sunday morning. Mash the feta into the sauce and break into the golden oozing yolks with toasted pitta. Store any leftovers in an airtight container in the refrigerator and warm in a pan when you're ready for another round.

1 tablespoon olive oil

1 red onion, finely chopped

1 red (bell) pepper, cored, deseeded and diced

2 garlic cloves, minced

1 tablespoon sun-dried tomato paste

1 heaped teaspoon smoked paprika

¼ teaspoon ground cumin

Pinch of dried chilli flakes

500g (generous 2 cups) passata
(puréed canned tomatoes)

150ml (⅔ cup) water

100g (3½oz) feta cheese

4 medium free-range eggs

Salt and pepper

Chopped parsley, to garnish

Pitta breads, toasted, to serve

- Heat the oil in a large frying pan with a lid. Add the onion with a pinch of salt and sweat for 5 minutes over a medium heat until it softens. Stir in the red pepper, garlic, sun-dried tomato paste, smoked paprika, cumin and chilli flakes.

- Continue to sauté for a few minutes, then pour in the passata and water. Let this mixture simmer and reduce for about 10 minutes.

- After the sauce has thickened, season it with salt and pepper. Place the feta in the centre of the pan and gently press the block into the sauce. Create 4 small wells in the sauce and crack an egg into each one. Add a sprinkle of pepper over the feta.

- Cover the pan with its lid and allow the dish to cook gently. The eggs are done when the whites have set but the yolks remain runny (or cook for longer if you prefer firmer yolks).

- Once cooked, remove the lid. Garnish with parsley and sprinkle pinches of salt and pepper over each yolk. Serve with a toasted pitta for each person.

Eggy Bread with Tomato Salsa

Serves 1

Time:
10 minutes

Macros:
Under 300kcal,
18g protein

Inspired by fond childhood memories, this recipe is a recreation of a favourite breakfast that my mum often made. Simple yet deeply comforting, it offers a perfectly balanced start to the day. While sourdough is a great choice, you can use any bread you fancy, and when it comes to toppings, don't hesitate to get creative – try it with avocado and smoked salmon, or wilted spinach and feta cheese.

2 medium free-range eggs

1 tablespoon milk

1 large slice of sourdough or bread of choice

Handful of cherry tomatoes

Small handful of basil leaves

Squeeze of lemon juice

Olive oil, for cooking

Salt and pepper

- In a shallow bowl, whisk the eggs and milk together with salt and pepper to taste. Soak the bread in the mix while you prep the salsa garnish, turning it over from time to time.

- Dice the cherry tomatoes, chop the basil and combine in a bowl. Add lemon juice, salt and pepper to taste.

- Heat a nonstick frying pan over a medium heat, and lightly brush it with olive oil. Lay the soaked bread in the pan and cook for 2–3 minutes on each side, until golden.

- Transfer to a serving plate and top with the fresh tomato-basil garnish.

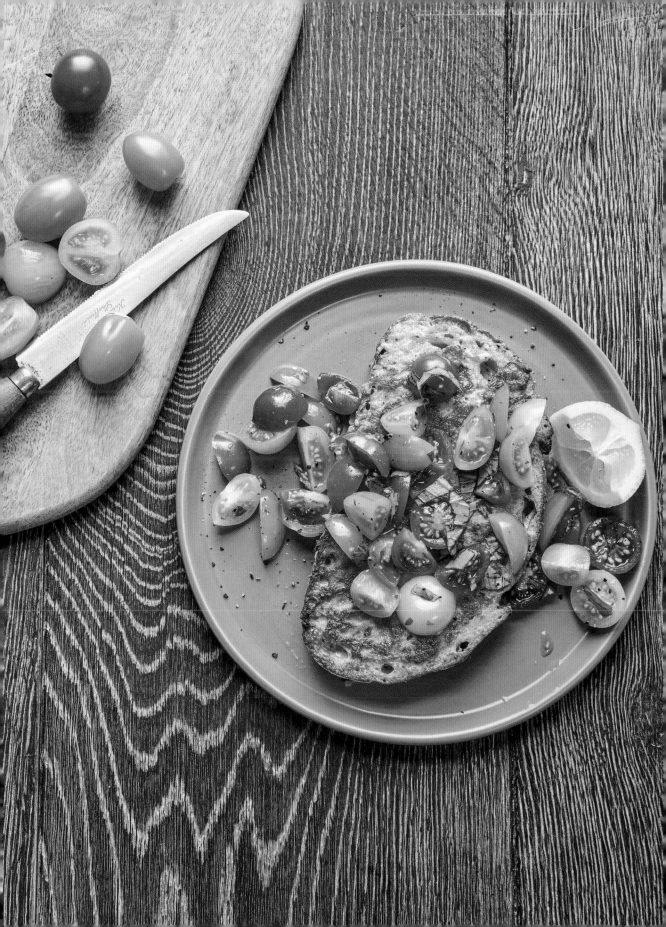

Hot Honey Halloumi Avocado Toast

Serves 2

Time:
15 minutes

Macros:
Under 450kcal,
22g protein per serving

One of my most popular recipes on social media, this Hot Honey Halloumi Avocado Toast is just the dream combination: toasted sourdough, crushed avocado, chopped parsley and lemon. Fry off your halloumi with a sticky and spicy honey-chilli mix and pair it with a 6-minute egg.

½ ripe avocado

2 tablespoons finely chopped parsley

Juice of 1 lemon

2 spring onions (scallions), finely chopped

4 teaspoons honey

2 teaspoons dried chilli flakes

2 medium free-range eggs, at room temperature

100g (3¼oz) halloumi cheese, sliced about 1cm (½ inch) thick

2 slices of sourdough or bread of choice

Salt and pepper

For the optional toppings

1 tablespoon finely chopped parsley

1 teaspoon dried chilli flakes

1 teaspoon honey

- In a bowl, mash the avocado and mix in the parsley, lemon juice and spring onion. Season with salt and pepper to taste, and set aside.

- In a separate small bowl, combine the honey, chilli flakes and a pinch of salt. Warm this mixture in the microwave on HIGH for about 15 seconds or until it turns runny.

- Fill a small pan with water and bring to a gentle boil. Carefully add the eggs and let them simmer for 6 minutes, then transfer to a bowl of iced water for 3 minutes. Once cooled, peel.

- While the eggs are cooking, fry the halloumi slices over a medium-high heat for about 2 minutes on each side, drizzling it with the honey-chilli mixture as you flip the slices occasionally, until the halloumi is golden brown and sticky.

- Meanwhile, toast your bread.

- Assemble your dish by first spreading the avocado mixture onto the toasted bread slices. Then top them with the sticky halloumi and any additional toppings, and place the halved soft-boiled egg on the side or on top of each slice, based on your preference.

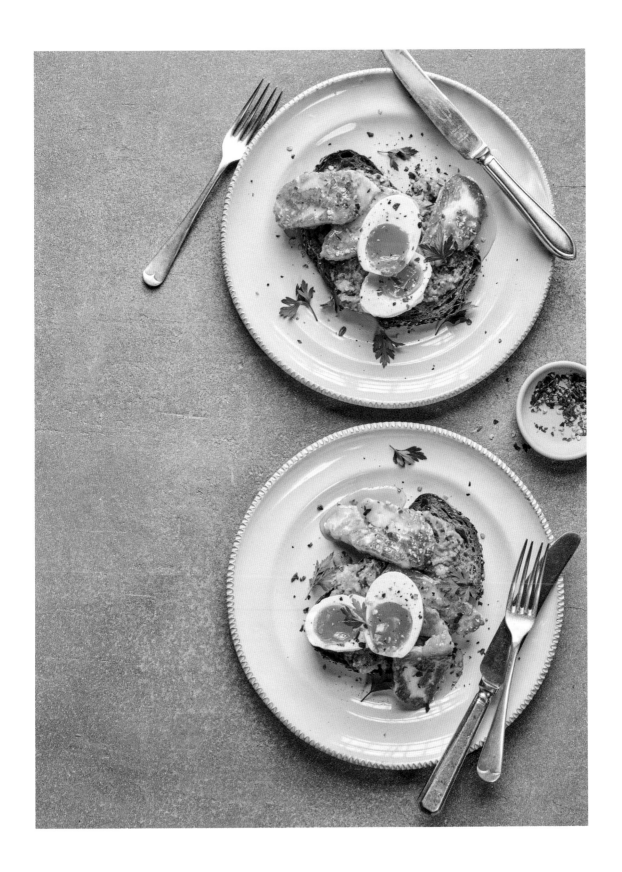

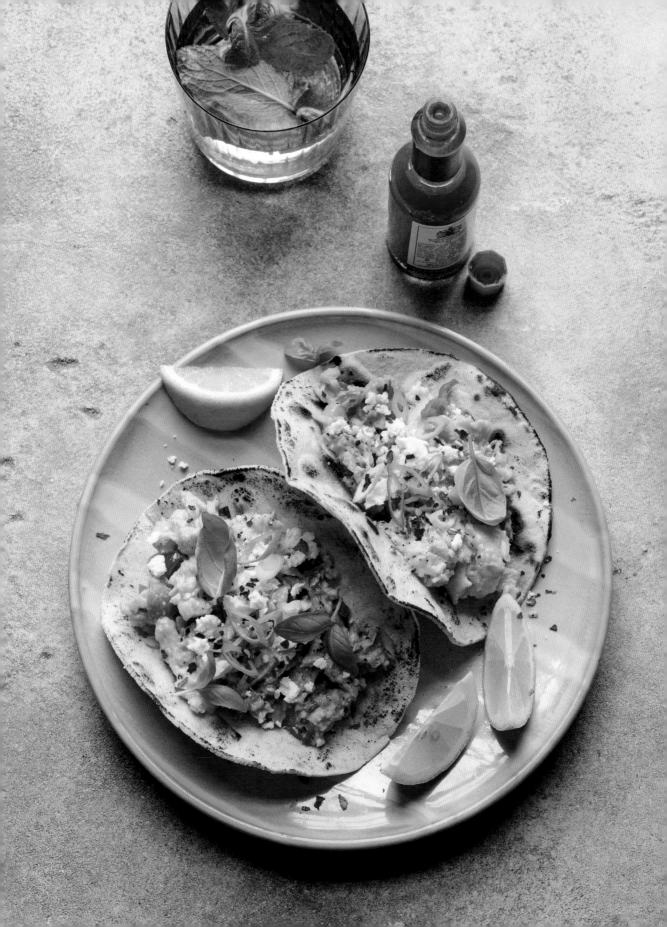

Morning Tacos

Serves 1

Time:
15 minutes

Macros:
Under 350kcal,
16g protein

These are so delicious and so quick too. I honestly could eat them for breakfast every day. The corn tortilla really makes these so I highly recommend you seek them out, but otherwise mini wheat tortillas will work fine. So simple, these will leave you feeling full, satisfied and balanced, plus they're great served with a dash of hot chilli sauce too.

¼ ripe avocado

1 spring onion (scallion), finely diced

Handful of cherry tomatoes, diced

Squeeze of lemon juice

Pinch of dried chilli flakes, plus extra to finish

5 basil leaves, chopped

2 medium free-range eggs

2 corn tortillas

10g (¼oz) feta cheese

Salt and pepper

For the optional toppings

1 tablespoon whole basil leaves

½ spring onion (scallion), finely diced

1 lemon, cut into wedges

- Begin by mashing the avocado in a bowl and then mixing with the spring onion, tomatoes, lemon juice, chilli flakes and basil. Season with salt and pepper to taste.

- In a separate bowl, whisk the eggs, adding a pinch of salt and pepper. Over a low heat, gently scramble the eggs in a nonstick pan.

- Toast your tortillas until lightly browned and crisp. Generously spread the avocado mixture over each, followed by a layer of scrambled egg. Finish by crumbling the feta over the top and adding an extra pinch of chilli flakes.

Prepable
Breakfast Muffins

Make a batch of these muffins and freeze them for an on-demand, healthy, convenient breakfast. The recipe features a superfood frittata and melty smoked cheese. Quick to prepare and easy to transport, they are a perfect speedy breakfast option.

Makes 4

Time:
15 minutes for frittata preparation, plus cooling and assembling time

Macros:
287kcal,
22g protein per muffin

2 medium free-range eggs

250g (9oz) fresh liquid egg whites (from a carton)

3 tablespoons chopped chives

Handful of chopped basil

1 red (bell) pepper, cored, deseeded and finely diced

1 tablespoon diced sun-dried tomatoes (roughly equivalent to 3–4 sun-dried tomatoes)

Olive oil, for greasing (if needed)

4 slices of smoked Applewood cheese (or use regular Cheddar)

4 English muffins (ideally wholemeal/wholewheat), cut in half

Salt and pepper

To serve *(optional)*

Sliced tomatoes

Baby spinach leaves

- Preheat the oven to 220°C/200°C fan (425°F) Gas Mark 7.

- In a bowl, whisk the whole eggs and egg whites together, then mix in the chives, basil, red pepper and sun-dried tomatoes. Season with salt and pepper and pour the mixture into a lined, oiled or nonstick baking dish, preferably 20 x 20cm (8 x 8 inches). This size will yield 4 muffin-sized squares that are around 2cm (¾ inch) thick.

- Bake the frittata in the oven for 5–10 minutes, or until just set. Allow it to cool completely in the dish/tin. This prevents breaking and sticking.

- Meanwhile, lightly toast the muffins.

- Cut the cooled frittata into 4 squares or circles. Place a slice of cheese on each square, sandwich each into a muffin, and wrap each sandwich in foil. These can be stored in the refrigerator for up to 3 days or frozen for up to 3 months.

- To serve, remove from the freezer and allow them to defrost overnight at room temperature.

- To heat, remove the foil and place each muffin on a microwave-safe plate. Microwave on HIGH for approximately 30 seconds, or until the centre is warm. Alternatively, heat the foil-wrapped muffins in a preheated oven at 180°C/160°C fan (350°F) Gas Mark 4 for 10–15 minutes.

- If desired, add in tomato slices and baby spinach leaves before serving.

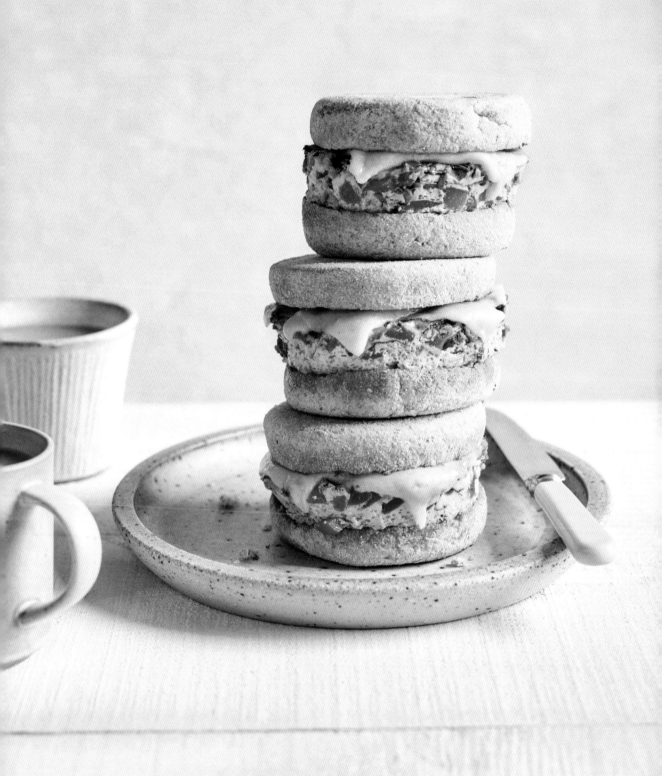

Crispy Feta Eggs

Serves 1

Time:
15 minutes

Macros:
Under 500kcal,
25g protein per serving

One of my favourite avocado toast combinations, the crispy salty feta pairs like a dream with the basil, tomato and avocado mixture spread onto warm sourdough. The crumbled feta melts into the pan and forms lovely crispy edges to the fried eggs. I sometimes make this for a quick lunch too!

1 ripe tomato, deseeded and diced

½ ripe avocado, peeled, stoned and diced

1 spring onion (scallion), finely sliced

A few basil leaves, chopped

½ teaspoon honey

Pinch of dried chilli flakes

1 slice of sourdough bread, about 60g (2¼oz)

30g (1oz) feta cheese

2 medium free-range eggs

Salt and pepper

- In a bowl, combine the tomato, avocado, spring onion, basil, honey and chilli flakes. Season with salt and pepper and roughly mash. Set to one side.

- Toast the sourdough.

- In a frying pan over a medium heat, sprinkle a circle of the feta, crack the eggs into the feta and fry until golden and crisp. I like to cover the pan with a lid to help the eggs cook on top without setting the yolks.

- Spread the avocado mix over the toasted sourdough, then serve with the crispy feta eggs. Season the egg yolks with an extra pinch of salt and pepper.

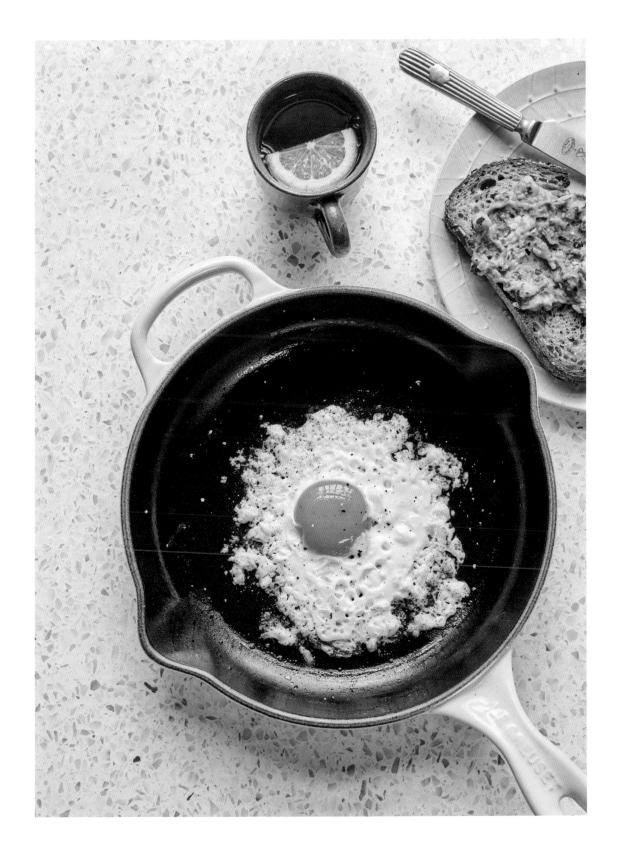

42-81

Lunch

42 Mango, Jalapeño and Lime Salad

46 Tuna Melt

49 Crunchy Peanut Slaw

50 Toasted Sesame and Ginger Chicken Salad

52 Speedy Chicken and Spicy Guacamole Tacos

55 Nature's Multivitamin

56 Best Ever Caesar Salad

58 Detox Gyoza Soup

61 Lighter Pesto Pasta Salad

62 Sushi Salad

64 Whipped Feta and Smoked Salmon Open-faced Sandwich

67 The Glow Bowl

68 Satay Salmon with Smacked Cucumber Salad

69 Egg 'Not Mayo' Sandwich

70 The 'I Have No Time' Tuna Salad

72 Oven-baked Feta and Pepper Pasta

75 Greek Salad-inspired Chicken Pittas

76 Skin Glow Omega Bowl

78 Sticky Honey Halloumi Salad

Mango, Jalapeño and Lime Salad

One of my favourite salads, this dish is full of glow-giving goodness and packed with flavour. It's everything you want in a meal and so simple to make. Roast your chickpeas with a coating of cornflour and spices until they are golden and crisp. The dressing, which uses jalapeño brine, adds a subtle warmth and flavour that is simply heavenly. Simply toss everything together and serve.

Serves 2

Time:
25 minutes, plus time for cooling

Macros:
Under 450kcal,
23g protein per serving

400g (14oz) can of chickpeas, drained, rinsed and dried

1 teaspoon cornflour (cornstarch)

1 teaspoon garlic granules

1 teaspoon smoked paprika

2 teaspoons olive oil

200g (7oz) ripe mango flesh, diced

1 medium ripe avocado, halved, stoned, peeled and diced

¼ cucumber, deseeded and diced

¼ red onion, thinly sliced

2 tablespoons diced jalapeños (from a jar)

150g (5½oz) cooked peeled prawns (shrimp), or substitute with tofu for a veggie option

2 large handfuls of chopped coriander (cilantro) or parsley

Salt

1 lime, cut into wedges to garnish (optional)

For the dressing

2 tablespoons jalapeño brine (liquid from the jar)

Juice of 1 lime

1 teaspoon honey

1 teaspoon Dijon mustard

- Preheat the oven to 230°C/210°C fan (450°F) Gas Mark 8, or set an air fryer to 200°C (400°F).

- In a mixing bowl, toss the chickpeas in the cornflour, garlic granules and smoked paprika, and season with salt. Drizzle in the olive oil and stir until the chickpeas are well coated.

- Spread the chickpeas in a single layer on a baking tray and roast in the oven or air fryer for 15–20 minutes, until crisp and golden. Set aside to cool.

- While the chickpeas are roasting, prepare the dressing. In a small bowl, whisk together the jalapeño brine, lime juice, honey and Dijon mustard, adding salt to taste. Check and adjust, adding more honey or lime juice as needed.

- In a large salad bowl, prepare your vegetables. Combine the mango, avocado, cucumber, red onion, diced jalapeños, prawns (or tofu), and coriander or parsley.

- Add the cooled roasted chickpeas to the salad bowl, pour over the dressing and toss everything together until well combined. Serve immediately.

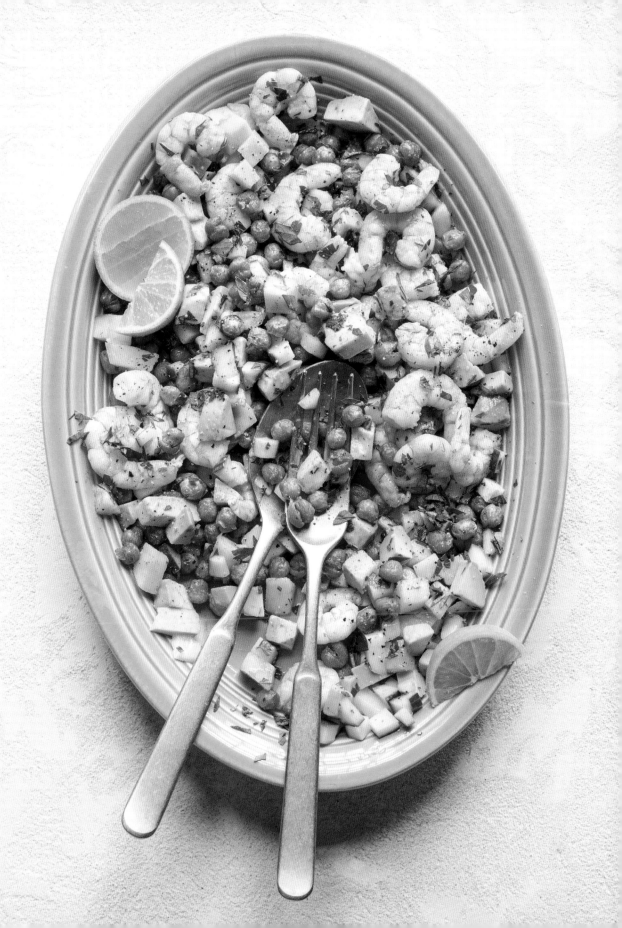

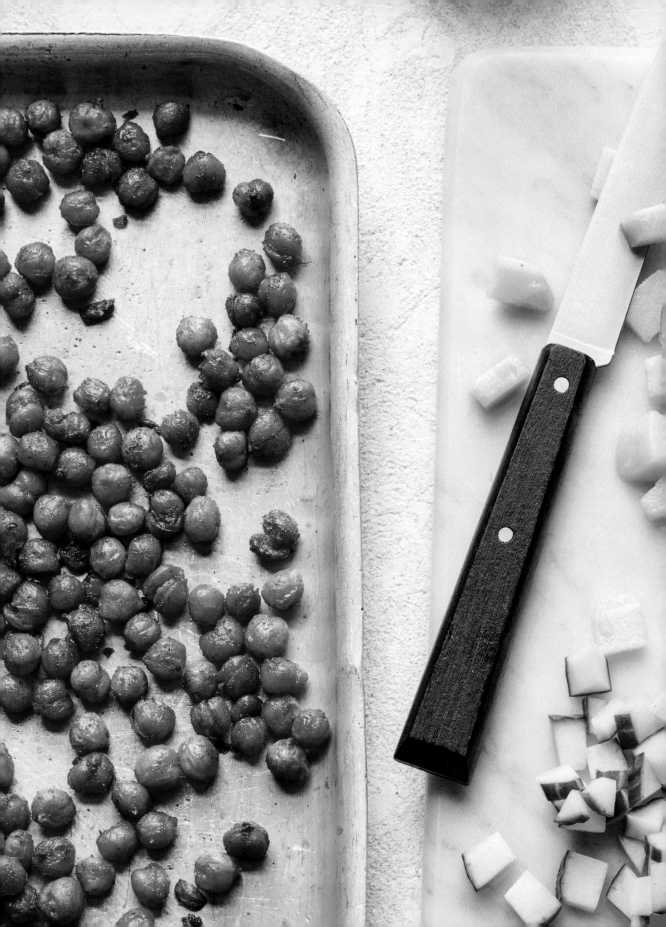

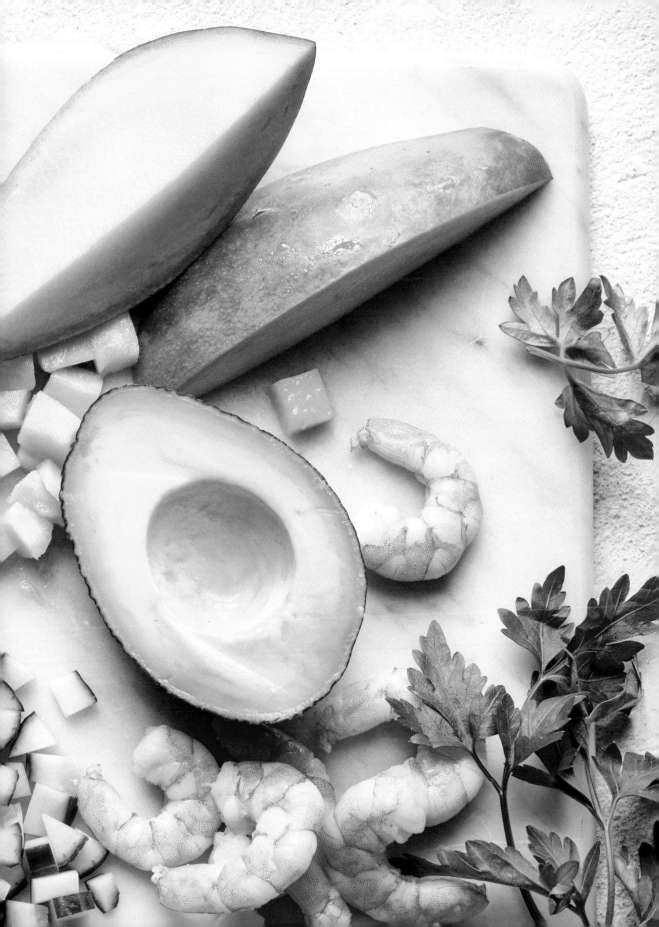

Tuna Melt

A tuna melt is undeniably comforting. One thing I love to do with these classic recipes is make a few swaps to transform something we all know and love into a meal with extra nutritional benefits. The bread is brushed with garlicky extra virgin olive oil for healthy fats, and the filling swaps mayo for a lighter, high-protein yogurt mix.

Serves 1

Time:
10 minutes

Macros:
Under 535kcal,
36g protein

60g (2¼oz) drained canned tuna in brine, flaked

1 spring onion (scallion), chopped

1 tablespoon capers, chopped

1 heaped tablespoon thick natural yogurt

1 teaspoon American mustard

1 teaspoon white vinegar

2 teaspoons extra virgin olive oil

1 garlic clove, finely chopped

Small handful of parsley leaves, finely chopped

2 slices of bread of choice

40g (1½oz) mature Cheddar cheese, grated

Salt and pepper

- In a bowl, mix the tuna with the spring onion, capers, yogurt, mustard and vinegar. Season with salt and pepper.

- In another small bowl, mix the olive oil with the garlic and parsley, and season with salt and pepper.

- Brush the garlic olive oil over both slices of bread on one side only. Flip the slices over and spoon the tuna mixture onto the un-oiled sides.

- Sprinkle the grated cheese over the tuna mix and press the sandwich together.

- Cook either in an air fryer at 200°C (400°F) for 3 minutes, flipping it over and cooking for a final 2 minutes until golden brown, or in a dry frying pan over a low-medium heat for a total of 5 minutes, flipping it so that both sides turn golden and the cheese melts.

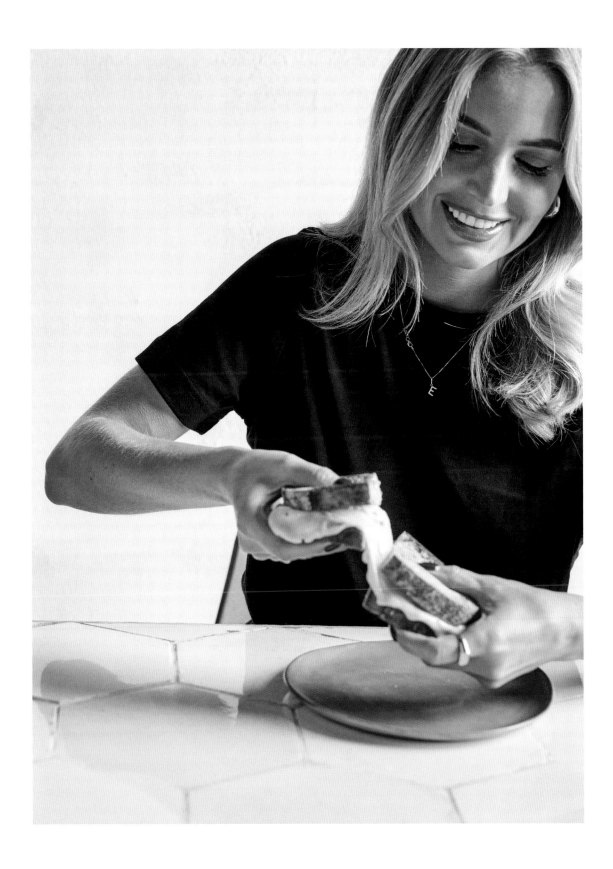

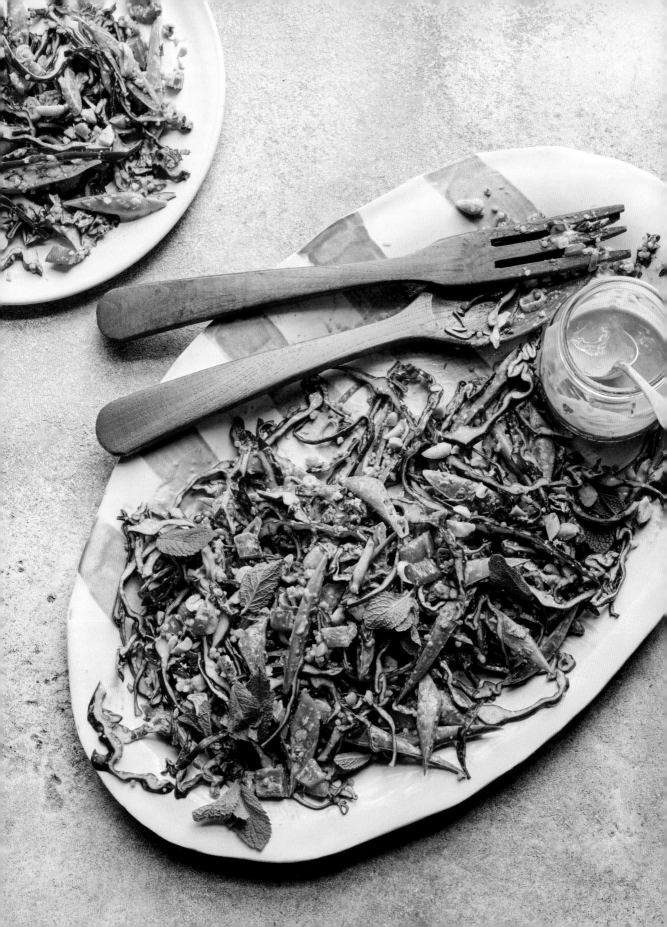

Crunchy Peanut Slaw

This is my Crunchy Peanut Slaw, packed full of freshness and glow-giving nutrition. The salad base will stay fresh for up to 3 days when stored in the refrigerator, making this an excellent choice for meal prep. Pair it with any protein of your choice to make this a quick, healthy and balanced lunch.

Serves 4

Time:
20 minutes

Macros:
For the salad base,
under 250kcal,
9g protein per serving

¼ red cabbage

50g (1¾oz) cooked quinoa or rice

2 cupped handfuls of sugar snap peas, sliced diagonally

3 spring onions (scallions), finely sliced

Large fistful of mint leaves

1 red (bell) pepper, cored, deseeded and diced

Small handful of roasted peanuts, roughly chopped

For the satay dressing

2 tablespoons smooth peanut butter

2 tablespoons light soy sauce

Juice of 2 limes

2 teaspoons ginger paste

2 teaspoons garlic paste

2 teaspoons honey

Pinch of salt

- Finely shred the cabbage: use either a swivel peeler to shave off super-thin shreds, or a mandolin or sharp knife for precise, thin shreds.

- Simply toss all the salad ingredients together in a bowl: shredded red cabbage, quinoa or rice, sugar snap peas, spring onions, mint leaves, red pepper and the roasted peanuts. Leave the salad unseasoned and undressed in an airtight container in the refrigerator for up to 3 days.

- Make the satay dressing by whisking the peanut butter, light soy sauce, lime juice, ginger paste, garlic paste, honey and a pinch of salt together in a small bowl or jar until smooth. If it is too thick, loosen with a little water. Season to taste with additional salt or soy sauce, as needed.

- To serve, pair the salad with a protein of your choice (such as grilled chicken, salmon, marinated tofu or prawns/shrimp), and generously drizzle the lovely satay dressing over the top.

Note:
It's important to leave the salad undressed if you're storing it for meal prep. Dress it only when you're ready to eat it to ensure that it stays fresh and crisp.

Toasted Sesame and Ginger Chicken Salad

This salad is absolutely delicious and strikes the perfect balance of crisp, crunchy, salty and fresh flavours. It's a protein powerhouse, with 56g per serving derived from a mix of both plants and chicken. This recipe is great for meal prep as it can be stored in the refrigerator for up to 3 days.

Serves 2

Time:
30 minutes, plus time for cooling

Macros:
Under 500kcal,
56g protein per serving

4–5 radishes, thinly sliced

150ml (⅔ cup) rice vinegar

2 teaspoons caster (superfine) sugar

100g (⅔ cup) frozen peas

150g (5½oz) cooked quinoa

¼ cucumber, deseeded and diced

2 spring onions (scallions), finely diced

½ ripe avocado, diced

1 roasted chicken breast, shredded

Handful of baby spinach leaves

Handful of coriander (cilantro), optional

For the roasted chickpeas

400g (14oz) can of chickpeas, drained, rinsed and dried

1 teaspoon toasted sesame oil

1 tablespoon light soy sauce

1 heaped teaspoon cornflour (cornstarch)

Pinch of salt

For the dressing

2 teaspoons ginger paste

2 teaspoons tahini

2 teaspoons toasted sesame oil

2 tablespoons light soy sauce

2 tablespoons rice vinegar

1 teaspoon honey

- Preheat the oven to 230°C/210°C fan (450°F) Gas Mark 8, or set an air fryer to 200°C (400°F).

- In a bowl, toss together the chickpeas with the toasted sesame oil, light soy sauce, cornflour and a pinch of salt. Spread the chickpeas in a single layer on a baking tray and roast in the oven or air fryer for 15–20 minutes, until crisp and golden. Set aside to cool.

- Meanwhile, place the radishes in a clean bowl and add the rice vinegar and sugar so the radish slices are completely submerged. Leave to pickle for at least 10 minutes. (Keep the leftover vinegar for future pickling projects!)

- Prepare the dressing in another bowl by whisking together the ginger paste, tahini, toasted sesame oil, soy sauce, rice vinegar and honey. Taste and adjust to your preference, adding more of any ingredient as needed.

- Cook the peas in a pan of boiling water for 2–3 minutes, or in the microwave according to packaging instructions, then drain.

- In a large salad bowl, toss together the roasted chickpeas, the quinoa, cucumber, spring onions, avocado, chicken, peas and drained pickled radishes. Add in the spinach, and the coriander, if using.

- Serve the salad in bowls with a generous drizzle of the dressing over the top.

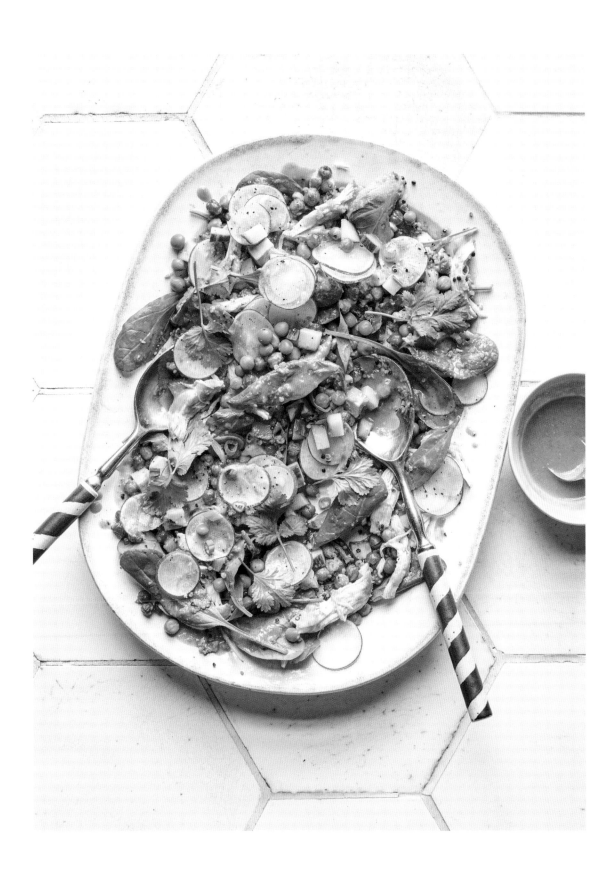

Speedy Chicken and Spicy Guacamole Tacos

Serves 1

Time:
15 minutes

Macros:
Under 450kcal,
20g protein

Quick and satisfying, these tacos are one of my go-to lunches. The pickled red onions will store for up to a month in the refrigerator. Pickles are a fantastic thing to include in your meals as they help with satiety and even blood sugar regulation. Swap the chicken for any protein of choice.

½ ripe avocado

1 teaspoon honey

1 spring onion (scallion), diced, plus extra to serve

3 jalapeños (from a jar), diced, plus 1 teaspoon brine from the jar

1 tablespoon chopped parsley

3 corn tacos

80g (2¾oz) cooked chicken breast, shredded

15g (½oz) feta cheese, crumbled

Salt

For the pickled onions

3 red onions, sliced into strips

White wine vinegar (enough to submerge the onions)

1 tablespoon caster (superfine) sugar

1 lime, cut into wedges, to serve (optional)

- For the pickled onions, add the red onion strips to a pan and pour in enough vinegar to completely submerge the onions. Add the sugar and gently heat to just before simmering, then take off the heat. Allow to cool slightly before use. Store any leftovers in a sealed jar or airtight container in the refrigerator for up to a month, for future use.

- In a bowl, mash the avocado and combine with the honey, spring onion, diced jalapeños and the brine, and the parsley. Season with salt to taste.

- Warm the tacos in a hot, dry frying pan on both sides.

- Begin by spreading the avocado mixture over each taco. Add the chicken, the feta, some (drained) pickled onions and some extra spring onion and lime wedges to finish. Serve immediately.

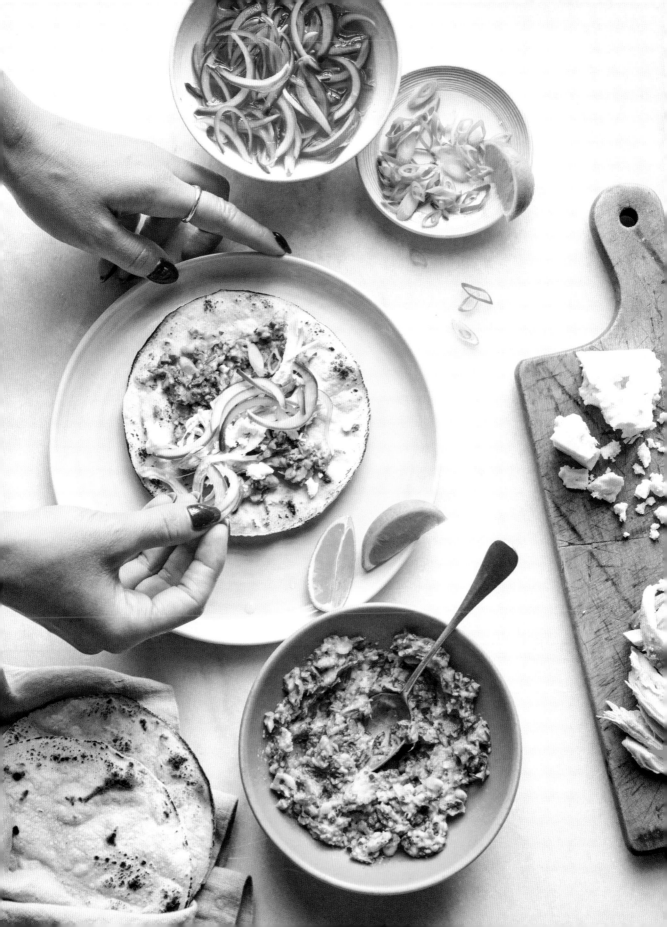

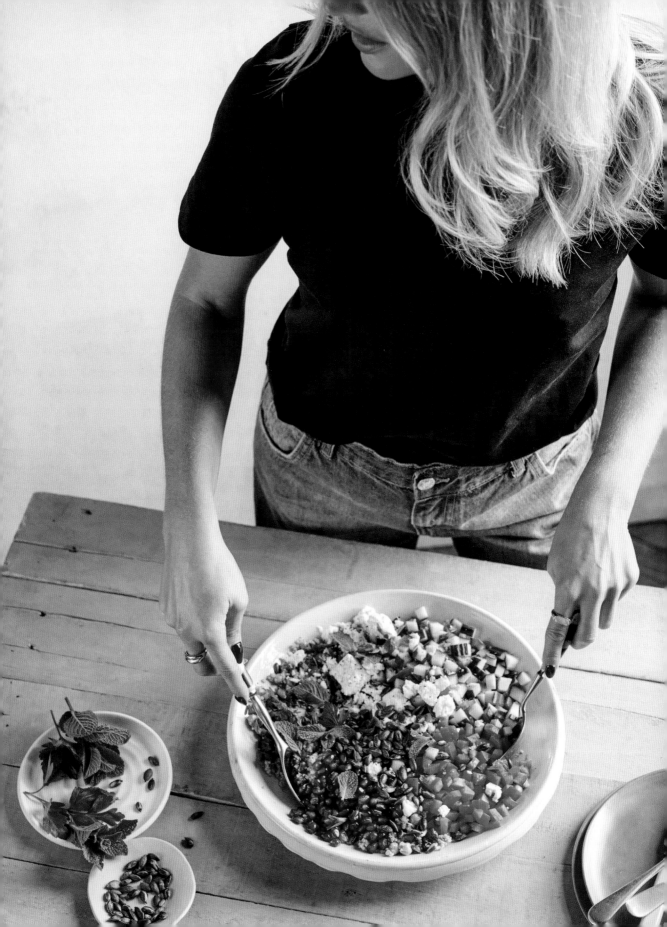

Nature's Multivitamin

Brimming with essential vitamins, minerals and antioxidants, I call this chopped quinoa salad Nature's Multivitamin because it really does contain everything we need to feel our best. Pumpkin seeds are a rich source of magnesium and give a gorgeous crunch to this salad. Leave undressed and store for up to 3 days in the refrigerator for leftovers, and pair with additional protein if desired.

Serves 4

Time:
15 minutes

Macros:
Under 300kcal,
9g protein per serving

2 tablespoons pumpkin seeds

½ cucumber

1 red (bell) pepper, cored, deseeded and diced

2 tablespoons capers

½ red onion, finely diced

80g (2¾oz) pomegranate seeds

Handful of mint leaves

Handful of parsley leaves

400g (14oz) can of chickpeas, drained and rinsed

250g (9oz) cooked quinoa

100g (3½oz) feta cheese

Salt and pepper

For the dressing

1 heaped teaspoon Dijon mustard

1 tablespoon extra virgin olive oil

Juice of 1 lemon

1 heaped teaspoon honey

- In a dry frying pan over a medium heat, lightly toast the pumpkin seeds for a few minutes, then season with salt, tip onto a plate and set to one side.

- Dice the cucumber, removing the seeds (this prevents the salad from going soggy).

- In a large mixing bowl, combine the cucumber, red pepper, capers, red onion, pomegranate seeds, mint, parsley and chickpeas. Fold in the cooked quinoa, crumble in the feta and sprinkle in the toasted pumpkin seeds.

- In a small bowl, whisk together the Dijon mustard, olive oil, lemon juice and honey until well combined, seasoning with salt and pepper.

- Drizzle the dressing over the salad, tossing gently to coat all the ingredients evenly.

- Serve immediately, or refrigerate for later.

Best Ever Caesar Salad

This iconic salad often gets a bad rep for its nutritional value. I have made this version for years now and it's one I come back to again and again; nothing beats it and I guarantee it will be one of the best Caesars you have ever made.

Serves 2

Time:
20 minutes

Macros:
Under 400kcal,
30g protein per serving

1 thick slice of sourdough, about 80g (2¾oz)

2 teaspoons extra virgin olive oil

1 sprig of thyme, leaves stripped

½ teaspoon garlic granules

3 slices of Parma ham

1 romaine lettuce, sliced

Handful of cherry tomatoes, halved

160g (5¾oz) cooked chicken breast, sliced

Salt and pepper

For the dressing

4 anchovies in oil

2 tablespoons thick kefir or strained natural yogurt

Juice of 1 lemon

15g (½oz) Parmesan cheese, grated, plus extra to serve

2–3 teaspoons Worcestershire sauce, to taste

¼ teaspoon garlic granules

- Preheat the oven to 190°C/170°C fan (375°F) Gas Mark 5.

- Cut the sourdough into cubes and toss in the olive oil, picked thyme leaves, garlic granules and salt to taste. Spread out in a single layer on an oven tray and bake in the oven for 15 minutes, turning occasionally, until golden.

- Meanwhile, pan-fry the Parma ham in a dry frying pan over a medium-high heat, turning a few times until lightly coloured. Allow it to cool on kitchen paper to turn crisp.

- Blend the dressing ingredients together in a food processor or blender. There's no right or wrong here; adjust it according to your taste. You might prefer more Worcestershire sauce and a strong lemon flavour. The dressing should have a loose consistency, not too thick. Add more yogurt to thicken if necessary and season with a few turns of black pepper.

- Assemble the salad in a bowl by combining the lettuce, tomatoes, chicken, crispy ham and a generous amount of the dressing. Mix everything well, then add the sourdough croutons and give it a final toss.

- Finish the salad with a grating of Parmesan, then serve.

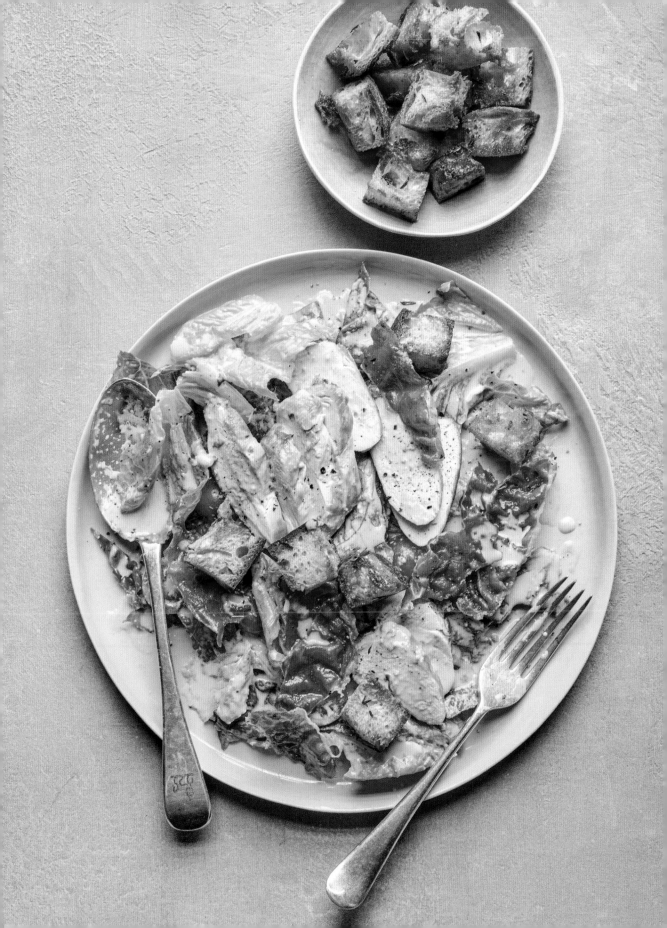

Detox Gyoza Soup

Serves 1

Time:
10 minutes

Macros:
Under 400kcal,
20g protein

There is nothing better than a comforting bowl of this Detox Gyoza Soup. It's quick and easy but also a nutritional powerhouse; an ideal choice for those who want to make a speedy but healthy lunch in just 10 minutes. I always have a packet of frozen gyoza in my freezer to rustle this one up and am always impressed at how delicious it is with such minimal effort.

300ml (1¼ cups) water

1 tablespoon light soy sauce

1 20g (¾oz) sachet of miso soup

1 carrot, peeled into ribbons

1 head of bok choy, base cut off

6 frozen gyoza (I use chicken)

1 egg

1 teaspoon crispy chilli oil

1 spring onion (scallion), finely sliced

- Add the water to a pan with the soy sauce and the contents of the miso soup sachet. Bring to a gentle simmer, then add the carrot and bok choy and simmer for 1 minute. Drop in the frozen gyoza and simmer for 3–4 minutes until the gyoza are cooked through.

- In a small bowl, whisk the egg, then slowly pour it into the hot soup, stirring gently to allow ribbons to form.

- Serve with the crispy chilli oil drizzled over, and a scattering of spring onion on top.

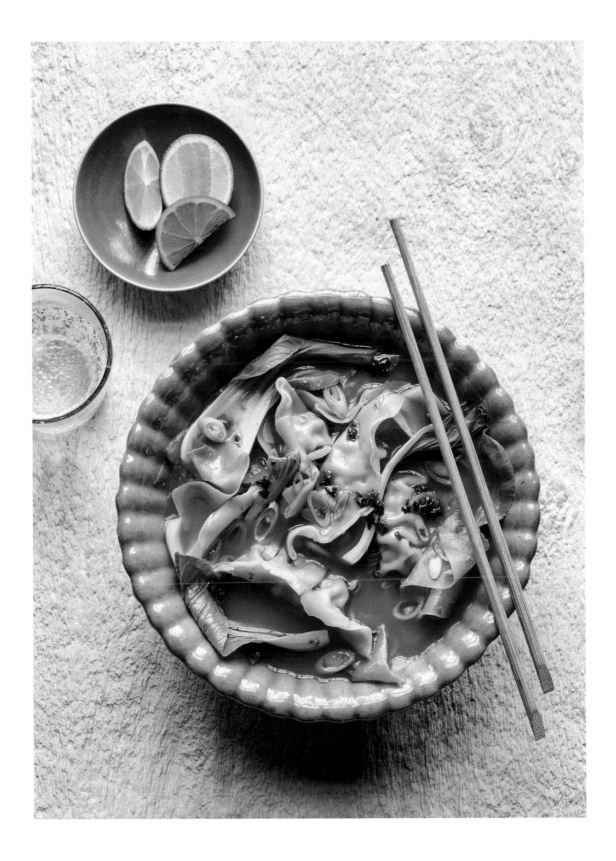

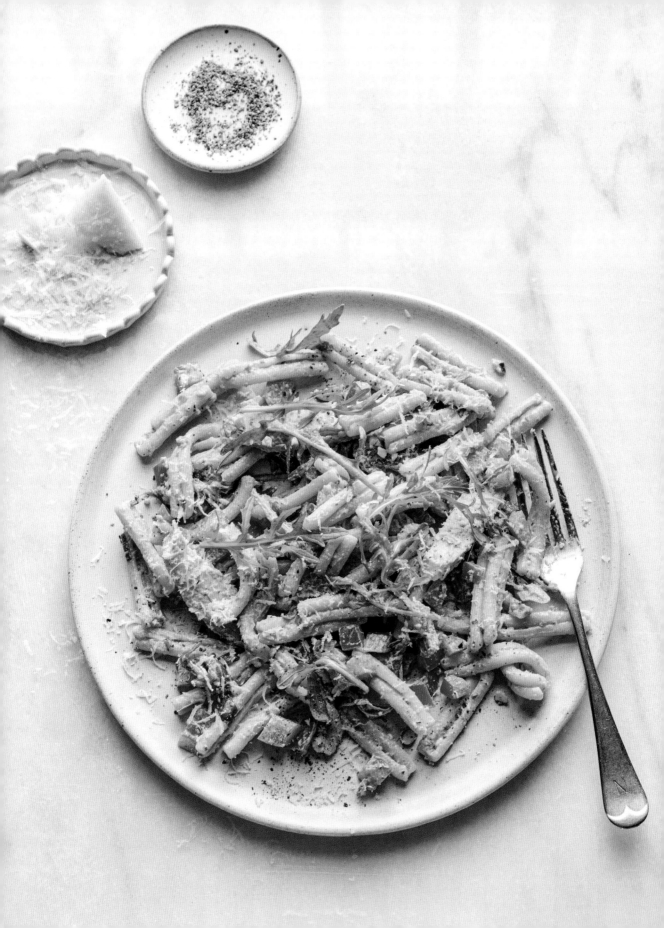

Lighter Pesto Pasta Salad

This is my take on a pesto pasta salad, one of my favourite lunches, but with a more balanced approach to ensure you are left feeling fuelled and satisfied. I have created a tangy pesto yogurt dressing full of fresh basil to toss through the pasta. Using fresh herbs in your meals is such an amazing way to pack in key vitamins and antioxidants. Simple but so delicious.

Serves 1

Time:
15 minutes

Macros:
Under 350kcal,
15g protein

---

1 large tomato, deseeded and diced

1 spring onion (scallion), finely chopped

A few basil leaves, roughly torn

Grating of Parmesan cheese, plus extra to serve

Pinch of dried chilli flakes

2 tablespoons thick natural yogurt (0% fat)

1 heaped tablespoon green pesto

1 teaspoon garlic paste

Zest and juice of 1 unwaxed lemon

60g (2¼oz) dried pasta of choice

80g (2¾oz) protein of choice, such as cooked chicken breast, sliced, or cooked peeled prawns (shrimp)

Handful of rocket (arugula) leaves

Salt and pepper

- In a bowl, combine the tomato, spring onion, basil, Parmesan and chilli flakes. Mix well and set aside.

- To make the pesto dressing, in another small bowl, mix the yogurt with the pesto, garlic paste and lemon zest and juice, and season with salt and pepper to taste. Whisk until well combined.

- Cook the pasta in a pan of boiling salted water, according to the packet instructions. When the pasta is cooked to your liking, drain, reserve 1–2 tablespoons of the pasta cooking water and add it to the bowl with the tomato mixture. Mix well.

- Pour the pesto dressing over the pasta, add the tomato mixture, and toss until everything is well coated and combined.

- Fold in your choice of protein and the rocket, ensuring they are well distributed throughout the salad.

- Serve the pasta salad with an extra flourish of freshly grated Parmesan on top.

Sushi Salad

All the flavours of sushi in a super simple and easy salad mix. Full of protein, healthy fats and fibre perfect for keeping you full and energised. The pickled radishes provide freshness as well as help balance blood sugar levels. Ideal for prepping, leftovers will keep for up to 3 days in the refrigerator. Feel free to swap the tuna for salmon, chicken or tofu.

Serves 2

Time:
15 minutes

Macros:
Under 450kcal,
15g protein per serving

100g (⅔ cup) frozen peas

1 medium ripe avocado, halved, stoned, peeled and diced

½ cucumber, deseeded and diced

2 spring onions (scallions), chopped

2 nori sheets, shredded, plus extra to serve

120g (4¼oz) drained canned tuna in brine

250g (9oz) packet of precooked brown rice (I use Tilda)

For the pickle

10 pink radishes

100ml (scant ½ cup) rice vinegar

100ml (scant ½ cup) water

1 heaped teaspoon caster (superfine) sugar

For the dressing

2 tablespoons light soy sauce

1 heaped teaspoon tahini

1 teaspoon wasabi paste

1 tablespoon mirin

- For the pickle, using a mandolin or sharp knife, thinly slice your radishes. Mix the rice vinegar, water and sugar together in a small pan. Warm on the hob or in the microwave on HIGH until just below simmering, then turn off the heat. Drop the sliced radishes into the pickling liquid and leave to one side.

- Cook the peas according to the packet instructions, drain and leave to one side to cool slightly.

- Mix the dressing ingredients together in a small bowl and set to one side.

- In a separate bowl, mix together the peas, avocado, cucumber, spring onions, shredded nori sheets and tuna. Tip in the packet of cold rice and a few spoonfuls of the drained pickled radishes, then toss through the dressing. Serve with extra nori on the side for scooping.

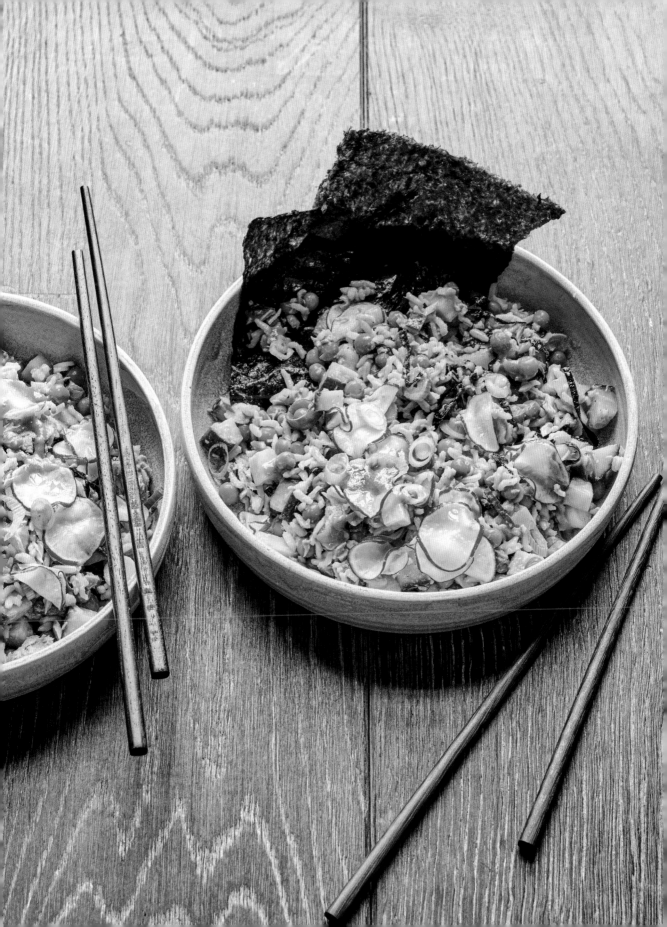

Whipped Feta and Smoked Salmon Open-faced Sandwich

Serves 1

Time:
15 minutes

Macros:
Under 350kcal,
20g protein

An open-faced sandwich is one of my favourite quick and easy lunches. The potential to load up a good slice of sourdough with healthy toppings is endless. This version uses creamy whipped feta and smoked salmon to provide a good source of protein and omega-3 fatty acids.

2 tablespoons thick strained natural yogurt (0% fat)

20g (¾oz) feta cheese

Zest of ½ unwaxed lemon, plus 1 tablespoon juice

5cm (2 inch) piece of cucumber, deseeded and diced

1 spring onion (scallion), finely sliced

1 tablespoon capers

1 slice of sourdough bread, about 60g (2¼oz)

50g (1¾oz) smoked salmon

Pepper

Small handful of dill leaves, to garnish (optional)

1 lemon, cut into wedges, to serve (optional)

- For the whipped feta, combine the yogurt and feta in a bowl and roughly mash using the back of a fork until you have a smooth consistency, being careful not to over-blend. Stir through the lemon zest and juice, and season with a little pinch of pepper.

- In a bowl, mix the cucumber, spring onion and capers together.

- Toast the sourdough, then spread the whipped feta cheese on top.

- Spoon the cucumber mixture over the whipped feta, then add ribbons of smoked salmon on top and garnish with the dill, black pepper and lemon wedges.

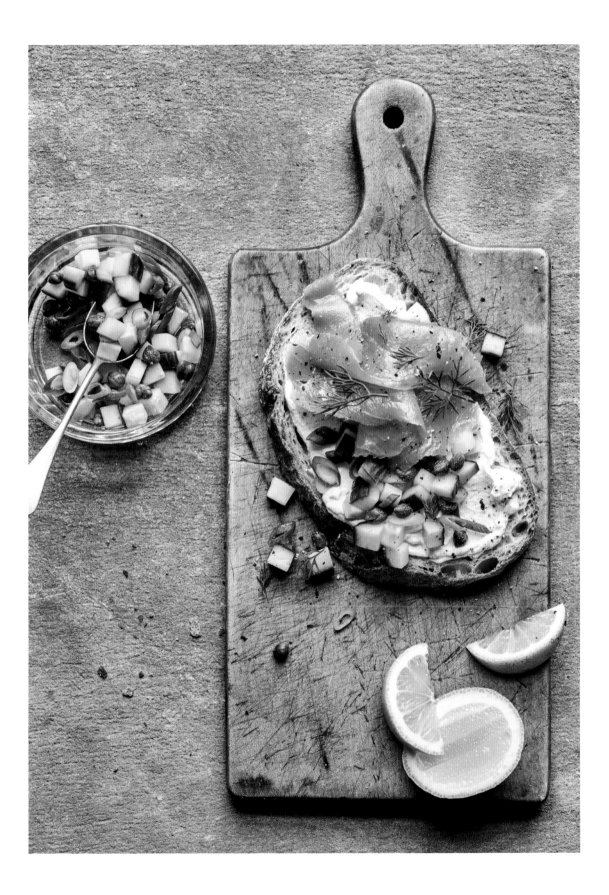

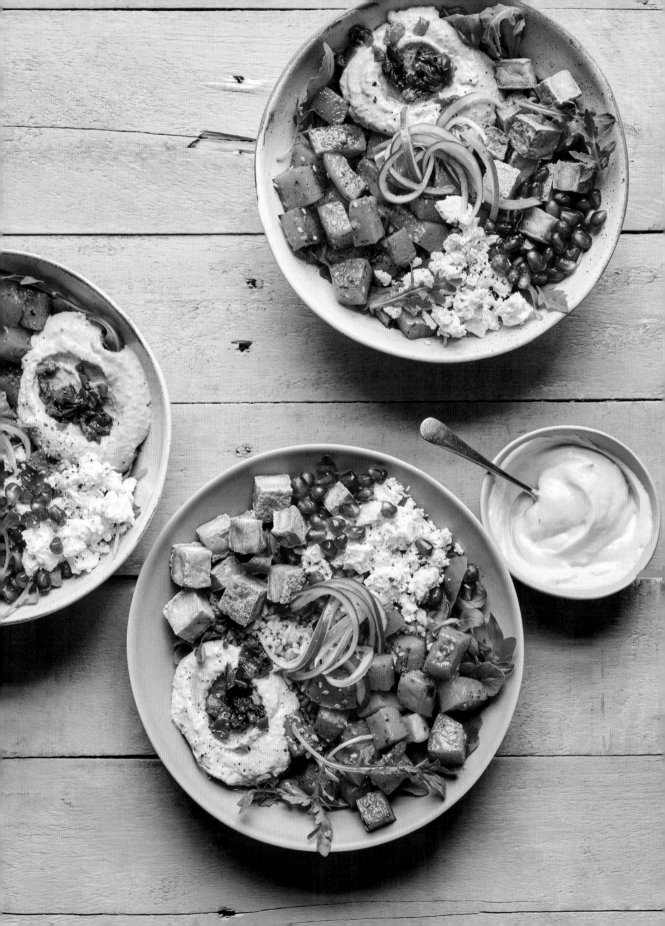

The Glow Bowl

Serves 4

Time:
35 minutes

Macros:
Under 400kcal per
serving, protein
depends on what
you use

Back in lockdown, I used to have a Deliveroo kitchen and my
Glow Bowl was one of my best sellers. A heavenly mix of grains,
feta, jalapeño hummus, roasted squash and pickled red onions.
It can be stored in the refrigerator for up to two days, and makes
great meal prep.

500g (1lb 2oz) peeled, deseeded butternut squash

1 tablespoon za'atar spice mix

1 tablespoon olive oil

1 jar of jalapeños

250g (9oz) cooked grain of choice

60g (2¼oz) rocket (arugula) leaves

200g (7oz) feta cheese, crumbled

200g (7oz) hummus

Protein of choice (cooked chicken, tofu, prawns/shrimp,
etc.)

80g (2¾oz) pomegranate seeds

Salt and pepper

1 lemon, cut into wedges, to serve

For the pickle

150ml (⅔ cup) white wine vinegar

100ml (scant ½ cup) water

1 tablespoon caster (superfine) sugar

2 red onions, sliced into rounds

For the dressing

150g (⅔ cup) natural yogurt

1 tablespoon tahini

Juice of 1 lemon

1 teaspoon honey

- For the pickle, pour the vinegar and water into
  a pan, add the sugar and bring to a simmer.
  Remove from the heat and immerse the red
  onion slices in the liquid. Let them pickle as you
  continue with the prep.

- Preheat the oven to 230°C/210°C fan (450°F)
  Gas Mark 8 or set an air fryer to 200°C (400°F).

- Cut the squash into 2cm (¾ inch) cubes and
  add to a heatproof bowl. Season with the za'atar
  spice mix and some salt and coat in the olive oil.
  Microwave on HIGH for 5 minutes, then spread out
  on a baking tray and either roast in the oven, or in
  the air fryer, for 10 minutes. Remove and set aside.

- In a bowl, mix the dressing ingredients (yogurt,
  tahini, lemon juice and honey) together with a
  pinch each of salt and pepper, and set aside.

- Make a jalapeño sauce by tipping the entire jar
  of jalapeños, including the brine, into a blender
  or food processor. Blend to achieve a chunky
  consistency. Store any leftovers in the original jar
  in the refrigerator, where it will last for a month.

- Microwave your chosen grains to heat through.

- Divide the rocket between 4 bowls, to create the
  base. Divide the grains, feta, roasted squash and
  hummus between the bowls. Create a well in
  the hummus using the back of a spoon and add
  1 teaspoon of jalapeño sauce to each. Add any
  extra protein of choice.

- Finish with the drained pickled red onions and the
  pomegranate seeds and serve with the dressing
  and lemon wedges.

Satay Salmon with Smacked Cucumber Salad

An easy midweek lunch when you're short on time. I simply adore these tangy smacked cucumbers tossed with soy sauce, rice vinegar, garlic and crispy chilli oil. They help keep you full, and balance your blood sugar. Feel free to pair this with a few spoonfuls of cooked rice or noodles.

Serves 2

Time:
45 minutes, including marinating

Macros:
Under 350kcal,
24g protein per serving

2 skinless salmon fillets

For the marinade

1 heaped tablespoon smooth peanut butter

1 teaspoon ginger paste

¼ teaspoon mild curry powder

2 tablespoons light soy sauce

1 tablespoon rice vinegar

1 teaspoon honey

For the smacked cucumber salad

1 cucumber

2 tablespoons rice vinegar

1 tablespoon light soy sauce

¼ teaspoon garlic granules

1 teaspoon caster (superfine) sugar

1 teaspoon crispy chilli oil

1 teaspoon salt

- Mix the marinade ingredients together in a bowl, add the salmon fillets and mix to coat. Cover and refrigerate for at least 30 minutes.

- Preheat the oven 230°C/210°C fan (450°F) Gas Mark 8, or set an air fryer to 200°C (400°F).

- Take the whole cucumber and, using a rolling pin, smack the cucumber so that it splits, then chop into 2cm (¾ inch) pieces.

- Put the cucumber into a mixing bowl with the rice vinegar, soy sauce, garlic granules, sugar, chilli oil and salt, toss together and leave to sit.

- Take the salmon from the refrigerator, mix into the marinade one more time, then place on a baking tray and bake in the oven or air fryer for 8 minutes until golden and the salmon flakes easily.

- Serve the salmon with the smacked cucumber salad.

Egg 'Not Mayo' Sandwich

An egg mayo sandwich is a fantastic high-protein and nutrient-rich lunch, but swapping the classic mayo mix for my yogurt version lightens it up while also adding extra protein and calcium with no compromise on flavour. You can batch make this filling and eat it for lunch during the week; it will keep for up to two days in an airtight container in the refrigerator.

Serves 1

Time:
15 minutes

Macros:
Under 350kcal,
25g protein

2 medium free-range eggs

1 heaped tablespoon natural yogurt

1 teaspoon American mustard

1 spring onion (scallion), finely sliced

1 tablespoon chopped parsley

1 tomato, deseeded and diced

2 slices of bread of choice

Small handful of baby spinach leaves

Salt and pepper

- Bring a small pan of water to the boil. Lower in the eggs and cook for 8 minutes. Drain, place in a bowl of iced water for 2 minutes, then remove and peel.

- While the eggs are cooking, in a bowl, mix the yogurt, mustard, spring onion, parsley, tomato, a good pinch of salt and a crack of black pepper.

- Roughly chop the eggs, add to the bowl and carefully mix to combine.

- Spread the egg mixture equally over the 2 slices of bread and add the spinach leaves on top. Sandwich together and enjoy!

The 'I Have No Time' Tuna Salad

A quick-fix solution for busy days, this salad delivers flavour and nutrition in just a few minutes. Swap the tuna for any protein of choice.

Serves 1

Time:
5 minutes

Macros:
Under 300kcal,
28g protein

145g (5¼oz) can of tuna in spring water, drained and flaked

¼ medium ripe avocado, diced

2 tablespoons drained canned chickpeas

Handful of rocket (arugula) leaves

Handful of cherry tomatoes, halved

1 tablespoon capers

20g (¾oz) feta cheese, crumbled

¼ cucumber, deseeded and diced

¼ red onion, finely diced

For the dressing

1 tablespoon natural yogurt

1 teaspoon American mustard

1 teaspoon honey

Juice of ½ lemon

Salt and pepper

- Combine all the ingredients in a bowl, including all the dressing ingredients, with salt and pepper to taste. Toss together and serve.

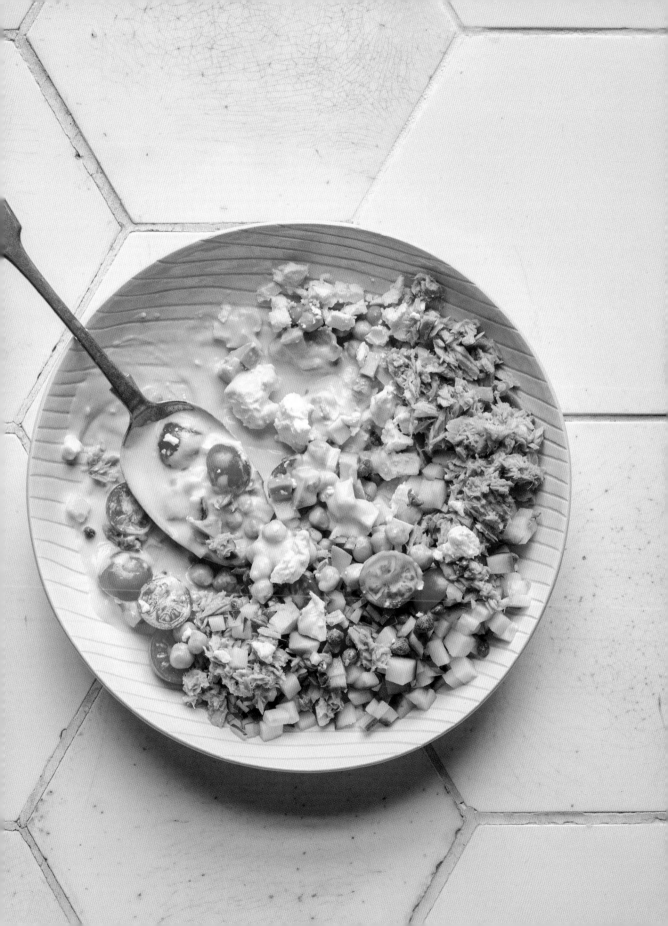

Oven-baked Feta and Pepper Pasta

Baking feta does something wonderful to it, intensifying the flavour and giving this pasta salad a special twist. Roast the red peppers in the same dish and simply mix with the cooked pasta and dressing. Boost the protein content by mixing through roasted chicken, cooked prawns (shrimp) or grilled/baked salmon.

Serves 4

Time:
35 minutes

Macros:
Under 450kcal,
15g protein per serving

150g (5½oz) feta cheese

1 large red (bell) pepper, cored, deseeded and sliced

1 large yellow (bell) pepper, cored, deseeded and sliced

1 tablespoon olive oil

1 tablespoon honey

Good pinch of dried oregano

250g (9oz) dried pasta of choice

½ red onion, finely diced

Handful of basil leaves

2 tablespoons capers

Small cupped handful of pitted green olives, halved

Salt and pepper

For the dressing

Juice of 1 large lemon

1 tablespoon white wine vinegar

1 heaped teaspoon Dijon mustard

1 heaped teaspoon honey

1 teaspoon garlic paste

- Preheat the oven to 230°C/210°C fan (450°F) Gas Mark 8.

- Place the block of feta in the centre of a baking dish or tray and scatter the sliced peppers around it. Drizzle over the olive oil and honey and sprinkle over the oregano and some salt and pepper. Bake in the oven for 25–30 minutes until golden.

- Meanwhile, cook the pasta in a pan of boiling salted water, according to the packet instructions. Drain and rinse under cold water to remove excess starch. Set aside.

- Mix together the dressing ingredients in a small bowl, seasoning with a pinch of salt.

- Combine the pasta, red onion, basil, capers, olives, roasted peppers, feta and dressing in a bowl. Add any extra protein at this stage, if you like. Toss well to break up the feta and coat the pasta, then serve.

- Store any leftovers in an airtight container in the refrigerator for up to 3 days, and enjoy cold or reheat in the microwave.

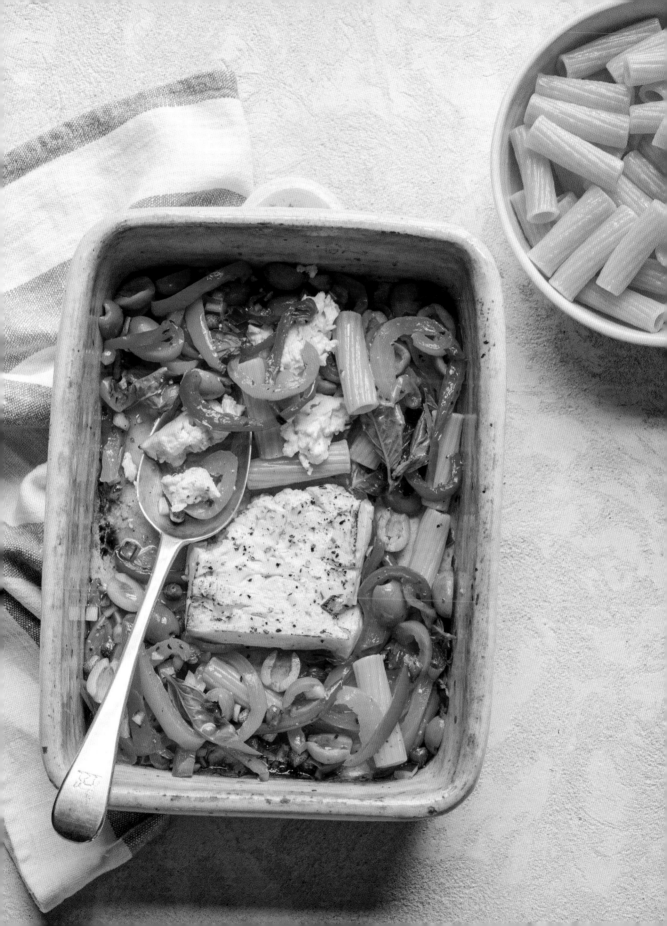

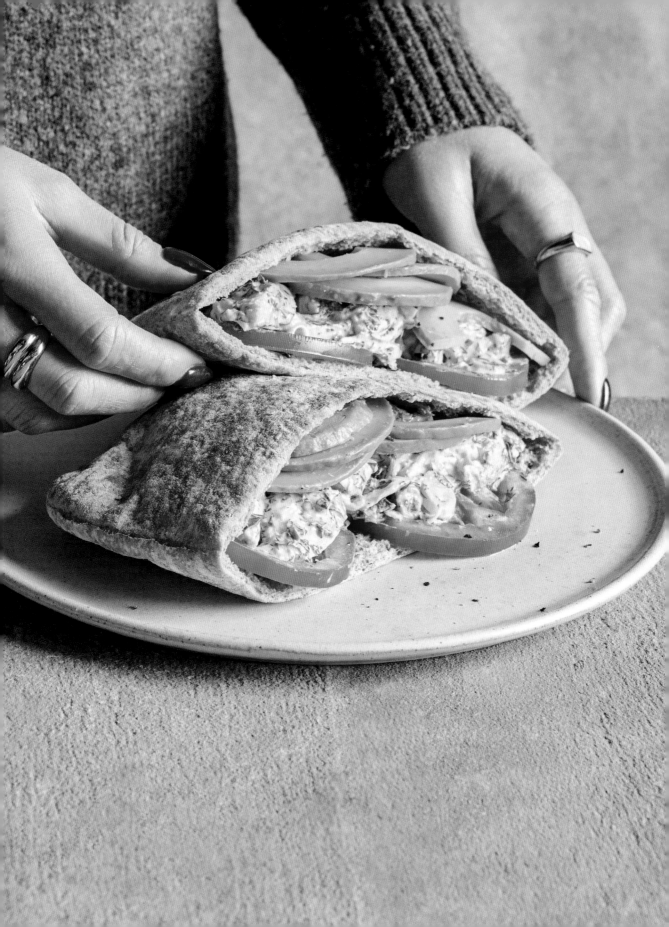

Greek Salad-inspired Chicken Pittas

Serves 1

Time:
10 minutes

Macros:
Under 400kcal,
30g protein

One of my favourite go-to lunches, this is both simple and delicious. It's the perfect solution for a quick lunch, requiring around 10 minutes to prepare. You can also pre-make the filling to streamline your weekly meals; it will keep in the refrigerator for up to 3 days. Don't hesitate to use this mix in wraps, or transform into a delicious sandwich.

80g (2¾oz) roasted chicken breast, shredded

1 tablespoon thick natural yogurt

Small handful of dill

Small handful of parsley leaves, roughly chopped

5 pitted black olives, diced

15g (½oz) feta cheese, crumbled

Zest of 1 unwaxed lemon and juice of ½ lemon

1 teaspoon American mustard

1 wholemeal (wholewheat) pitta bread

1 tomato, sliced

¼ ripe avocado, sliced

Salt and pepper

- In a bowl, combine the chicken, yogurt, dill, parsley, olives, feta and the lemon zest and juice. Add the mustard and season with salt and pepper.

- Warm the wholemeal pitta in a toaster, and then cut it in half, gently opening up the halves to create pockets.

- Stuff the pitta pockets with the chicken mixture, adding slices of tomato and avocado, then serve.

Skin Glow Omega Bowl

This salad is jam-packed with skin-supporting fats, omega-3s and antioxidants – perfect for giving you the glow. You can swap out mackerel for smoked salmon to suit your preference.

Serves 2

Time:
25 minutes

Macros:
Under 350kcal,
17g protein per serving

2 garlic cloves, unpeeled and smashed

350g (12oz) salad potatoes, cut into bite-sized pieces

2 spring onions (scallions), finely chopped

20g (¾oz) basil leaves, roughly chopped

Zest of ½ unwaxed lemon, plus 2 lemon wedges, to serve

2 tablespoons thick natural yogurt

1 teaspoon mild mustard

Handful of baby spinach leaves

½ cucumber, cut into thin rounds

140g (5oz) smoked mackerel fillets, skin removed

Salt and pepper

- Bring a pan of salted water to the boil. Carefully add the garlic cloves and potatoes to the boiling water, then bring back to a gentle simmer and cook for 10–15 minutes or until the potatoes are tender; check with a fork.

- Drain the potatoes, removing the garlic, and return them to the warm pan. Add the spring onions, basil, lemon zest, a pinch of salt and a crack of black pepper. Mix in the yogurt and mustard, tossing to combine.

- To serve, place a bed of spinach leaves in each bowl. Add the potato salad, arrange the cucumber rounds over the potato salad and then flake over the mackerel. Serve with a lemon wedge on the side.

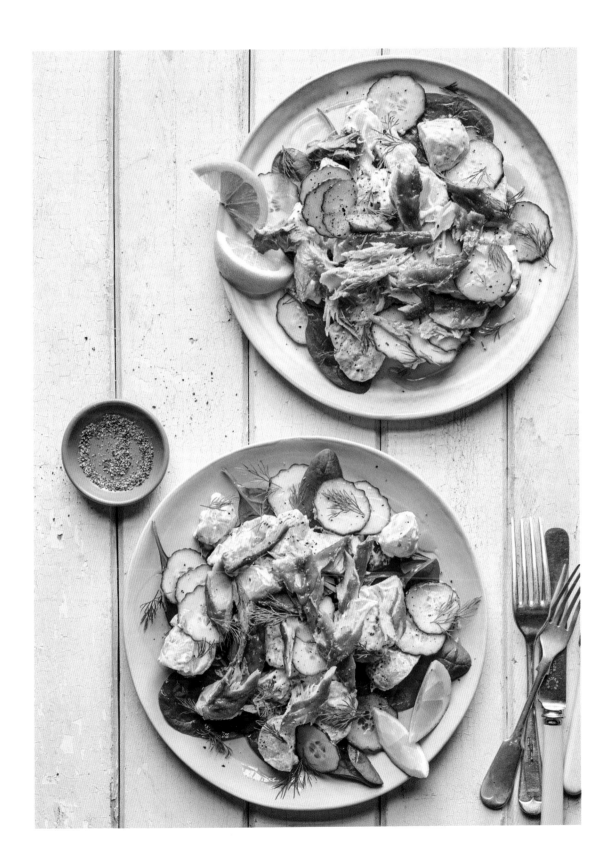

Sticky Honey
Halloumi Salad

Serves 4

Time:
30 minutes

Macros:
Under 400kcal,
20g protein per serving

Gone are the days of limp, unsatisfying salads. I'm going to show you how to create some of the most delicious and balanced salads that you will be eating on repeat. This is one of my signature salads: sweet and salty slices of pan-fried halloumi paired with roasted sweet potato and chickpeas, with the most delicious dressing packed with super-green goodness. Leftovers make great lunches – keep the undressed salad in the refrigerator for up to 2 days and the dressing will store for up to a week.

400g (14oz) can of chickpeas, drained, rinsed and dried

200g (7oz) sweet potato (unpeeled), diced into roughly 2cm (¾ inch) cubes

2 teaspoons cornflour (cornstarch)

1 teaspoon garlic granules

1 teaspoon olive oil

½ cucumber

2 handfuls of parsley leaves, roughly chopped

80g (2¾oz) pomegranate seeds

225g (8oz) halloumi cheese, cut into slices 1cm (½ inch) thick

1 teaspoon honey (for glazing halloumi)

Pinch of dried chilli flakes

Salt and pepper

For the dressing

2 tablespoons tahini

Handful each of chives, basil leaves and parsley leaves

½ teaspoon garlic granules

1–2 tablespoons lemon juice

1–2 teaspoons honey

2–3 tablespoons water

1 tablespoon pomegranate seeds (optional)

- Preheat the oven to 230°C/210°C fan (450°F) Gas Mark 8 or set an air fryer to 200°C (400°F).

- Coat the chickpeas and sweet potato in the cornflour, garlic granules and a generous pinch each of salt and pepper. Drizzle over the olive oil and mix to coat. Spread out in a single layer on a baking tray and roast in the oven or air fryer for 15–20 minutes until golden. Remove and set aside to cool a little.

- Meanwhile, place all the dressing ingredients in a blender or food processor, season with salt and pepper and blend until smooth, adding the lemon juice and honey to taste, and enough water for it to reach the right consistency. If it's too thick, simply loosen it with more water.

- Dice the cucumber, removing the seeds to prevent the salad from becoming soggy. Combine the diced cucumber with the parsley, pomegranate seeds and the crispy chickpeas and sweet potato on a platter.

- Fry the halloumi in a dry frying pan over a medium-high heat for 2 minutes, then add the honey and chilli flakes. Keep flipping every so often until the halloumi is evenly golden and sticky.

- Lay the halloumi slices over the salad, and drizzle over the vibrant green dressing to serve.

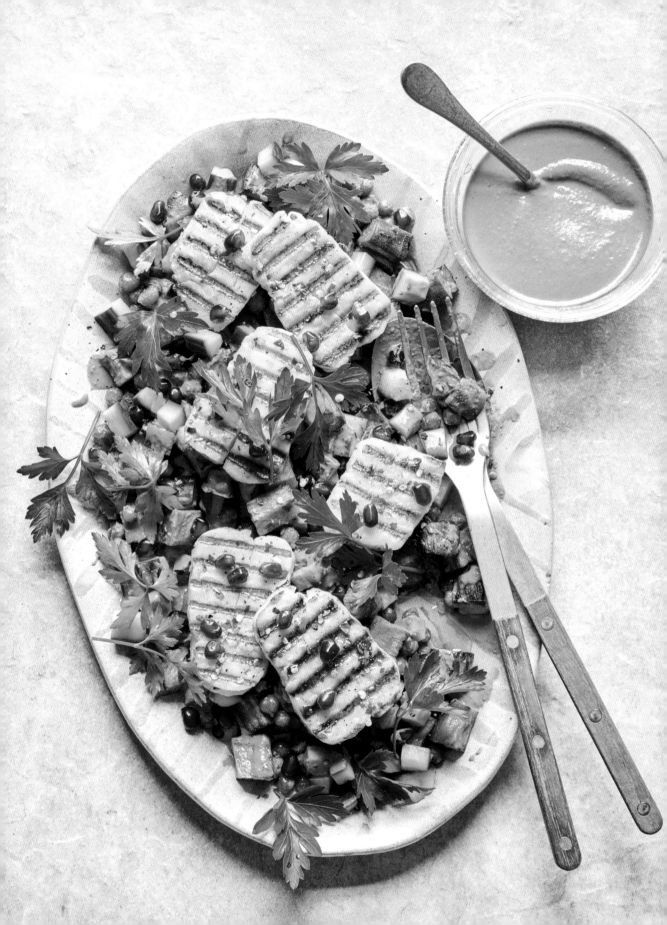

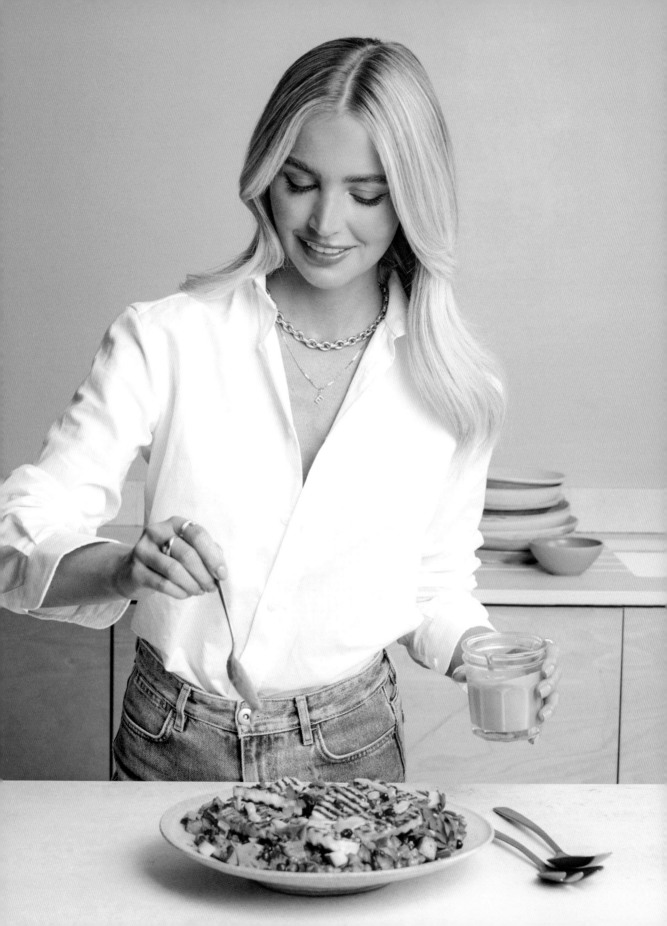

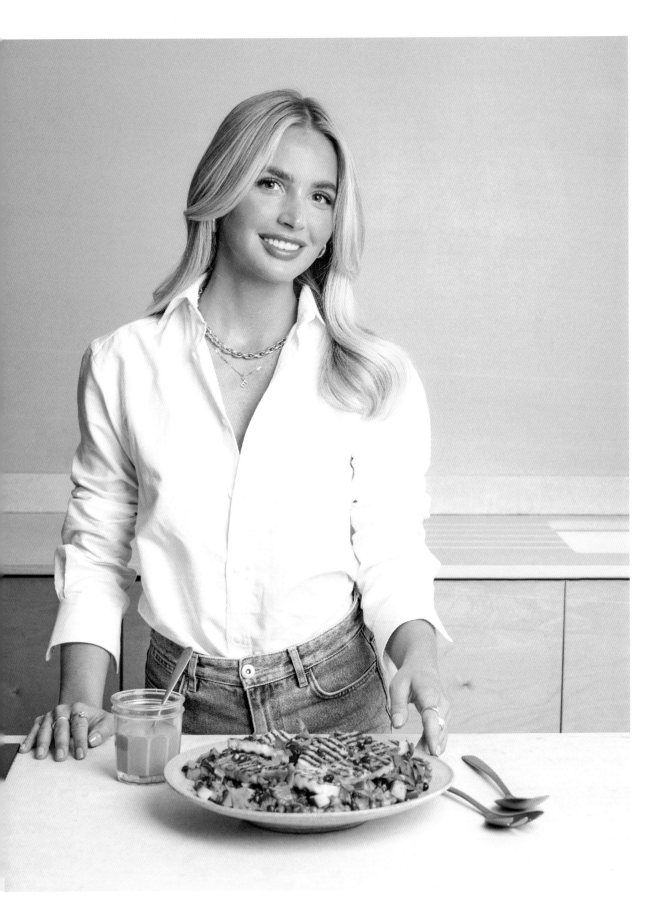

84-95

Snacks

84 Caramelised Onion Hummus

84 Beetroot and Mint Dip

85 Protein Power Pea and Bean Dip

88 Skin Glow Crackers

89 Smacked Cucumbers

89 Spicy Pepperoni Pizza Crispbread

90 Chicken Sausage Rolls

91 Super Seeded Chicken Nuggets
with Garlic Yogurt

94 Frozen Raspberry 'Popcorn' Yogurt Pot

95 Dark Chocolate Roasted Almond Bites

Caramelised Onion Hummus

Hummus has always been one of my favourite dips and this is my super-simple lighter hummus recipe that doesn't compromise on texture and flavour. If you can get your hands on the chickpeas in the glass jars, I highly recommend you do – they are so creamy and just take this recipe to the next level.

Serves 4

Time:
5 minutes

Macros:
Under 92kcal,
4g protein per serving

400g (14oz) can of chickpeas, drained and rinsed, reserving a little of the liquid from the can

1 heaped tablespoon tahini

1 tablespoon caramelised onion chutney

¼ teaspoon garlic granules

4 tablespoons jalapeño brine from a jar, or the juice of ½ lemon

Large pinch of salt

- Make the hummus by blending together the chickpeas, tahini, chutney, garlic granules, jalapeño brine or lemon juice, and a large pinch of salt. Add the reserved chickpea liquid to loosen as you blend, until you have a thick smoothie consistency. Taste and adjust if needed.

- Store in an airtight container in the refrigerator for up to 5 days.

Beetroot and Mint Dip

A vibrant but incredibly Moorish dip that is perfect for snacking with crudités, spreading over toast and even putting into sandwiches. Full of antioxidants as well as key nutrients for our skin health, this dip will leave you glowing.

Serves 4

Time:
5 minutes

Macros:
Under 88kcal,
9.5g protein per serving

250g (9oz) packet of cooked beetroot

1 tablespoon extra virgin olive oil

50g (1¾oz) feta cheese

Juice of ½ lemon

½ teaspoon garlic granules

1 tablespoon roughly chopped mint leaves

Salt and pepper

- Using a blender or a food processor, simply blitz the beetroot with the oil, feta, lemon juice, garlic granules, mint and some salt and pepper to taste until smooth.

- Store in an airtight container in the refrigerator for up to 4 days.

Protein Power Pea and Bean Dip

Serves 4

Time:
10 minutes

Macros:
Under 100kcal,
7g protein per serving

I love to batch make dips and spreads for simple, healthy snacking, and this is one of my favourite high-protein dips. Creamy cannellini beans, cottage cheese and peas blend into a thick and vibrant dip. Flavoured with fresh basil, Parmesan and lemon, it nods to all the flavours of pesto. Eat it like you would a hummus!

150g (1 cup) frozen peas

100g (¾ cup) drained canned cannellini beans

3 tablespoons cottage cheese

Handful of basil leaves

Zest of ½ unwaxed lemon

½ teaspoon garlic granules

15g (½oz) Parmesan cheese, grated

1 teaspoon honey

Good pinch each of salt and pepper

- Bring a pan of water up to the boil, add the peas and cook for 3 minutes, then drain well. Place in a blender with all the remaining ingredients and blend until smooth but still with a little texture.

- Store in an airtight container in the refrigerator for up to 4 days.

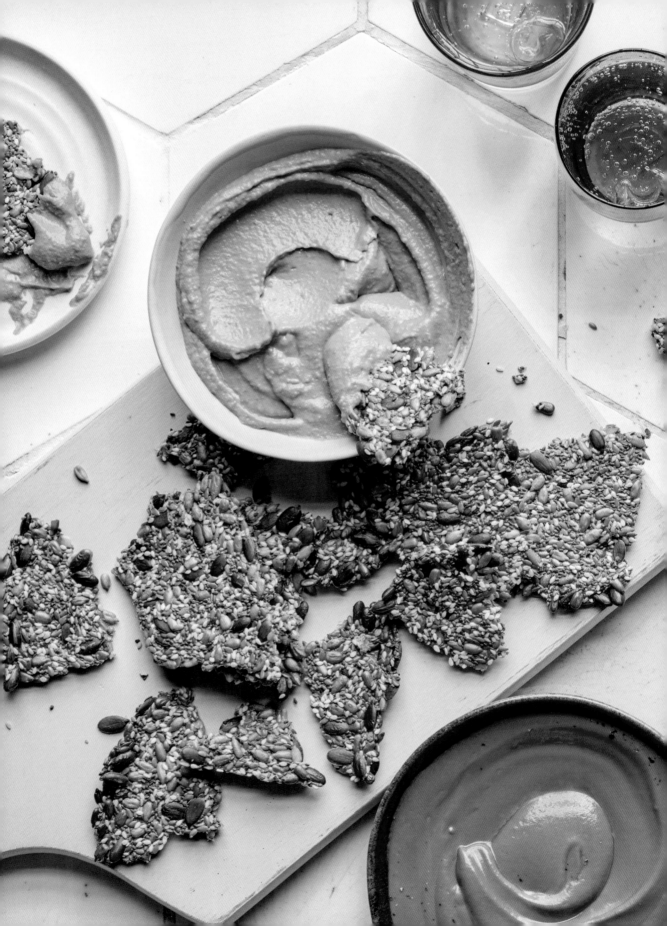

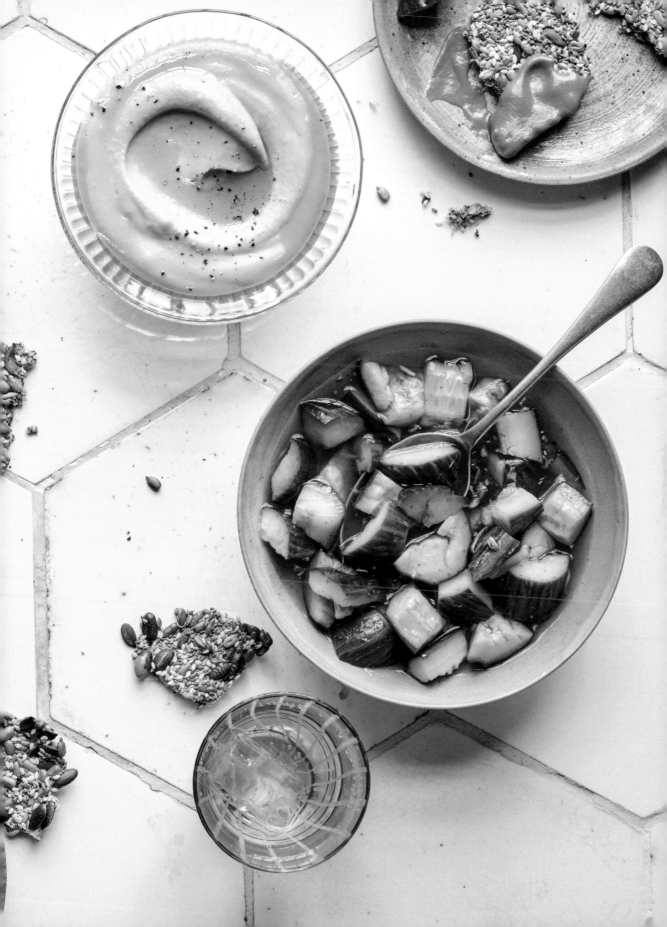

Skin Glow Crackers

Makes 20 portions

Time:
1 hour

Macros:
Under 150kcal,
5g protein per serving

Packed with a mix of nutrient-dense seeds, these crackers are a powerhouse of healthy fats, fibre and protein. Ideal for promoting healthy skin, they're a satisfying snack that pairs well with any dip, offering a healthful crunch that your body will thank you for.

160g (1⅓ cups) sunflower seeds

100g (¾ cup) pumpkin seeds

90g (½ cup) chia seeds

75g (½ cup) sesame seeds

60g (½ cup) whole flaxseeds (linseeds)

1 teaspoon za'atar spice mix

2 teaspoons flaky sea salt

400ml (1⅔ cups) warm water

- Preheat the oven to 200°C/180°C fan (400°F) Gas Mark 6. Line 2 large baking trays with nonstick baking paper.

- Combine all the seeds and the spice mix in a large bowl with the salt and warm water, and mix well. Leave to sit for 15 minutes, mixing every 5 minutes until the seeds soak up the water and the seed mixture becomes thick and gloopy.

- Spread the soaked seed mixture onto each lined baking tray around 0.5cm (¼ inch) thick. Bake in the oven for 45–60 minutes, until golden brown and crisp all over.

- Remove from the oven and allow the crackers to cool completely on the trays. Break into pieces and store in an airtight container for up to 7 days, perfect for dunking and dipping.

Smacked Cucumbers

Serves 4

Time:
10 minutes

Macros:
Under 50kcal,
5g protein per serving

I love to incorporate spicy pickled snacks into my diet as a great way to help satisfy cravings, balance my blood sugar and leave me feeling full. Once made, these cucumbers only get better and better as they sit and marinate during the week. You can store them in an airtight container in the refrigerator for up to 7 days.

1 large cucumber

80ml (⅔ cup) rice vinegar

1 tablespoon sriracha sauce

1 teaspoon honey

1 tablespoon light soy sauce

- Using a heavy rolling pin, hit the cucumber so that it splits, then chop it into bite-sized chunks.

- In a separate bowl, mix together the rice vinegar, sriracha, honey and soy sauce, then toss the cucumber chunks in the mix.

Spicy Pepperoni Pizza Crispbread

Serves 1

Time:
10 minutes

Macros:
Under 250kcal,
13g protein

The perfect light bite with all the flavours of a slice of pepperoni pizza: bright tomato sauce, oozy mozzarella and punchy pepperoni. These ingredients always bring a smile to my face when I get the afternoon nibbles. Feel free to swap the pepperoni for any of your favourite pizza toppings. The spice and chilli in these little crispbreads helps boost feelings of satiety to leave you feeling full.

2 tablespoons tomato pizza sauce of choice

2 crispbreads of choice (I like Ryvita)

30g (1oz) mozzarella pearls, torn

4 pepperoni slices, diced into small pieces

1 teaspoon diced jalapeños (from a jar)

Pinch of dried oregano

- Preheat the oven-grill to medium.

- Spread the pizza sauce over the crispbreads. Top with the torn mozzarella pearls, then evenly distribute the pepperoni and jalapeño pieces on top.

- Finish each crispbread with the oregano. Place under the grill until the mozzarella has melted and the pepperoni is golden, then serve.

Chicken Sausage Rolls

My take on a sausage roll makes the best high protein and portable snack. These snacks can survive any train or car journey, and are perfect for popping in your bag or bringing to picnics. With added courgette and chilli, these little rolls are full of fibre and flavour too. Super simple to make, you can store them in an airtight container in the refrigerator for up to 5 days.

Makes 16

Time:
20 minutes

Macros:
Under 100kcal,
7g protein per roll

500g (1lb 2oz) chicken sausagemeat or chicken mince

1 small red chilli, deseeded and diced

4 tablespoons chives, finely chopped

1 teaspoon ground black pepper

1 small courgette (zucchini), grated

1 medium free-range egg

270g (9¾oz) sheet of ready-rolled filo pastry

Olive oil spray

- Preheat the oven to 200°C/180°C fan (400°F) Gas Mark 6 or set an air fryer at 200°C (400°F).

- In a large bowl, combine the mince with the chilli, chives, pepper and grated courgette.

- Whisk the egg in a separate bowl and set aside.

- Unroll the filo and cut the large sheet in half so you have 2 pieces. Using an oil spray, spritz each filo layer to seal together.

- Halve the sausagemeat. Shape one portion into a long tube in the middle of one piece of filo sheet and roll up, leaving a 1cm (½ inch) section of filo at the end. Brush this section with egg and then finally seal to form a long roll. Repeat with the remaining sausagemeat and the second piece of filo sheet.

- Use a sharp knife, slice the long rolls into smaller 5cm (2-inch) rolls – there should be around 16 smaller rolls in total. Brush each smaller roll with the egg wash and a little extra pepper. Transfer to a lined baking tray.

- Bake in the oven or air fry for 15–20 minutes, until golden and cooked all the way through. Remove from the oven and leave to cool on the baking tray, or transfer to a wire rack until cooled.

Super Seeded Chicken Nuggets with Garlic Yogurt

Serves 4

Time:
25 minutes

Macros:
Under 200kcal,
20g protein per serving

Homemade chicken nuggets are simply the best. I boost these little bites by using a high fibre wholegrain and seeded crumb to coat the chicken before baking. Serve with a tangy garlic yogurt for a crowd-pleaser of a snack. You can prep and cook these, store in an airtight container in the refrigerator for up to 4 days and reheat when you need.

2 slices of seeded bread

½ teaspoon garlic granules

3 tablespoons plain (all-purpose) flour

2 medium free-range egg whites (I like to use fresh cartoned whites)

300g (10½oz) boneless, skinless chicken breast, cut into even nugget-sized pieces

Olive oil spray

Salt and pepper

For the garlic yogurt

150g (⅔ cup) thick natural yogurt (0% fat)

1 teaspoon white wine vinegar

1 teaspoon garlic granules

½ teaspoon dried oregano

1 teaspoon honey

- Preheat the oven to 210°C/190°C fan (410°F) Gas Mark 6½.

- Using a food processor or blender, blitz the bread and garlic granules into breadcrumbs.

- Create 3 bowls, one with seasoned plain flour, one with the lightly beaten egg whites and one with the breadcrumbs. Toss the chicken pieces in the seasoned flour, then into the egg whites, and then into the breadcrumbs, until evenly coated. Tip the coated chicken pieces onto a baking tray, spray with a little oil and then bake in the oven for 15 minutes, turning over halfway through, until golden and crisp.

- Meanwhile, to make the garlic yogurt, mix the yogurt with the vinegar, garlic and oregano. Add the honey and season with salt and pepper.

- Serve the crispy chicken nuggets with the garlic yogurt on the side.

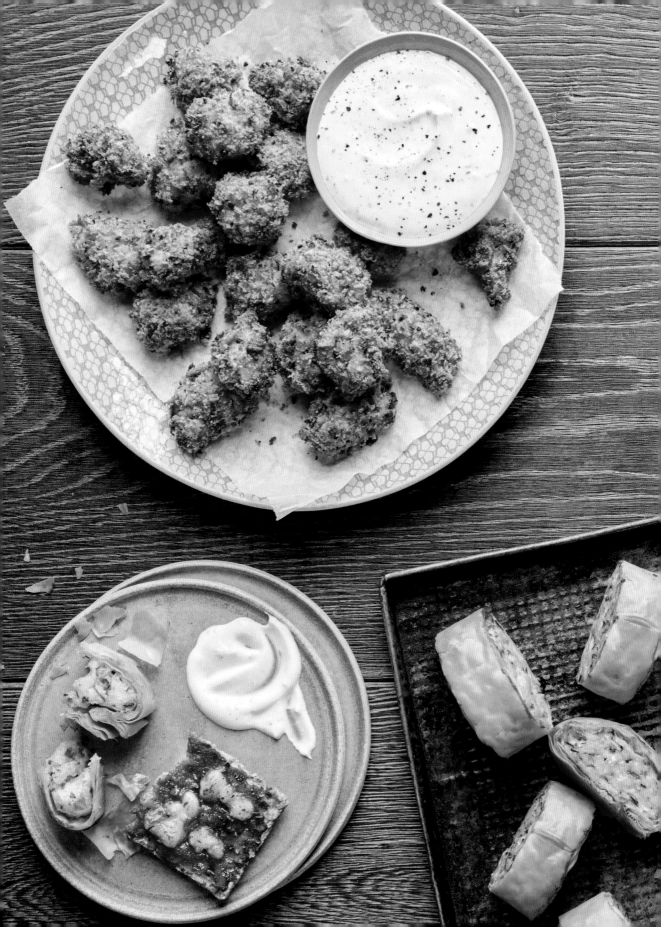

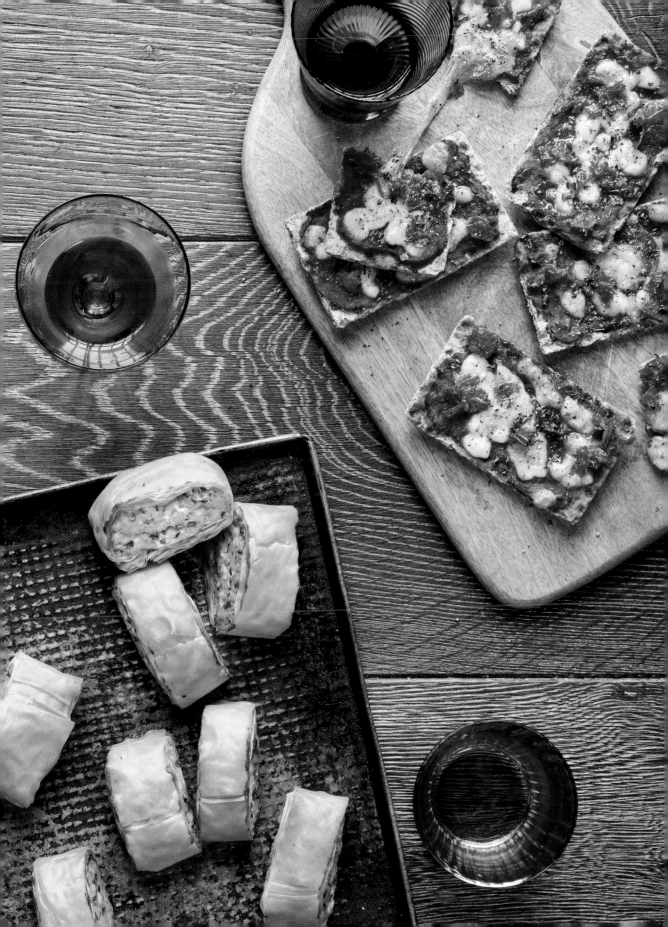

Frozen Raspberry 'Popcorn' Yogurt Pot

Serves 1

Time:
10 minutes

Macros:
Under 200kcal,
19g protein

This yogurt bowl is more a throw-it-all-together method than a recipe, but this combination has always been one of my favourite healthy snacks. Crushing up rice cakes into the frozen raspberry and yogurt mix gives the flavour of popcorn, paired with honey and crunchy toasted almonds, for the ultimate dessert. The combination of protein and fibre in this is a blood sugar balancing dream too, avoiding those unwanted spikes and crashes. Perfect to satisfy a sweet tooth.

6 skin-on whole almonds, roughly chopped

150g (⅔ cup) thick natural yogurt (opt for 0% fat to make this lighter)

30g (1oz) frozen raspberries, crushed

1 rice cake

1 teaspoon honey

- In a dry frying pan, toast the almonds over a low heat until they start to colour and smell nutty. Remove to a plate and set to one side.

- In a pot, mix together the yogurt with the crushed frozen raspberries. Crumble in the rice cake and mix, then top with a drizzle of honey and the toasted almonds.

Dark Chocolate Roasted Almond Bites

Makes 16

Time:
20 minutes

Macros:
Under 70kcal,
2g protein per serving

My favourite simple homemade chocolate bites, I used to serve these in my Deliveroo kitchen and they sold out every day. Toasting the almonds makes all the difference and gives these bites the most amazing flavour. Don't worry about them being perfectly uniform; there's something about the homemade look that adds to their charm. High in antioxidants and vitamin E too!

100g (¾ cup) skin-on whole almonds

100g (3½oz) dark chocolate (70% cocoa content), broken into pieces

Flaky sea salt

- Preheat the oven to 200°C/180°C fan (400°F) Gas Mark 6.

- Spread the almonds out on a baking tray and roast in the oven for 7–10 minutes, until they start to smell nutty and gorgeous. Avoid burning them, but make sure they are nicely toasted. Set to one side to cool.

- Lay a sheet of nonstick baking paper on a tray.

- Place the chocolate in a heatproof bowl and set it over a pan of simmering water (a bain-marie), making sure the base of the bowl isn't touching the water. Melt the chocolate, stirring until smooth, then mix in the cooled roasted almonds.

- Using 2 teaspoons, drop 16 bite-sized portions of the mixture onto the parchment-lined tray. Do this quickly before the chocolate sets.

- While the chocolate is still melted, sprinkle each bite with a pinch of flaky sea salt.

- Place in the refrigerator to set. Store in an airtight container in the refrigerator for up to a week.

98   Butternut Squash Mac and Cheese

100   Prawn and Sriracha Burgers

102   Pesto Prawn Courgetti Linguine

105   Brick Almond Chicken with Honey and Lime Slaw

106   My Best Ever Chicken and Tarragon Lasagne

108   Garlic-crumbed Salmon with Courgettes and Yogurt

111   Tuna Puttanesca Spaghetti

114   Chicken and Greens Pot Pie

116   'Ratatouille' Orzo with Sea Bass

118   Sticky Peanut Stir Fry

121   One-pan Tuscan Salmon

122   Meatball and Ricotta Al Forno

124   Smoky Mexican Black Bean Soup

125   Fish Pie with Garlic and Parmesan Crumb

126   Salmon and Sexy Veg

129   Spinach and Ricotta Malfatti

98–165

Dinner

130 Creamy Coconut Thai Green Noodles

132 Superfood Vegetarian Bolognese

135 Individual Salmon en Croûte

136 Chicken Katsu Curry

139 Chicken and Smoky Romesco

142 Wholegrain Fish and Chips with Tartare Sauce

146 Roasted Tomato Soup with Giant Parmesan Croutons

150 Creamy Parmesan Chickpeas with Pickled Chilli

152 Italian Sausage and Broccoli Pasta

156 Thai Chicken and Butternut Soup

158 Spiced Turkey Koftas with Tabbouleh and Mint Yogurt

163 Hot and Sour Thai Bowl

164 Harissa Roasted Red Pepper Immunity Soup

Butternut Squash Mac and Cheese

Who doesn't love a mac and cheese, a comfort food favourite that has received my signature glow up, using an extra virgin olive oil and Parmesan-spiked béchamel and sweet roasted butternut squash, a fantastic source of vitamin A. This dish was a top seller in my Deliveroo kitchen. Pair it with a simple salad for a fulfilling meal.

Serves 4

Time:
1 hour

Macros:
Under 500kcal,
21g protein per serving

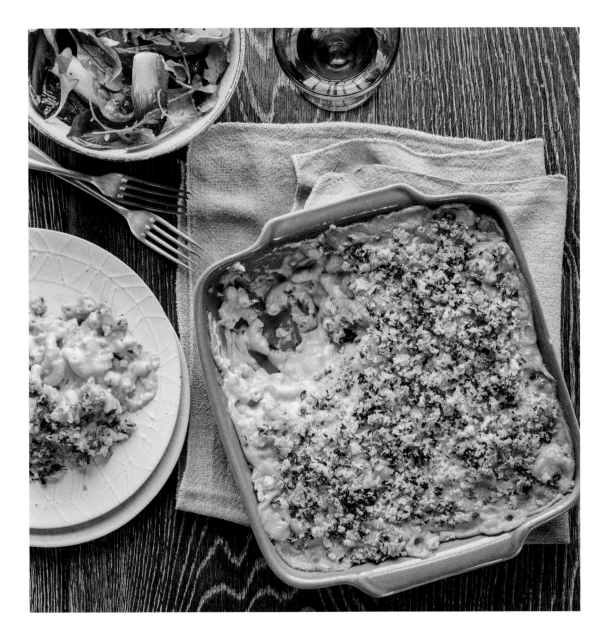

1 large butternut squash, halved lengthways and deseeded

1 tablespoon extra virgin olive oil, plus extra for drizzling

50g (1¾oz) sourdough bread

200g (7oz) dried macaroni

1 heaped tablespoon plain (all-purpose) flour

600ml (2½ cups) semi-skimmed milk

30g (1oz) Parmesan cheese, grated

50g (1¾oz) extra-mature Cheddar cheese

1 chicken stock cube, crumbled

1 tablespoon American mustard

Small handful of parsley leaves

½ teaspoon garlic granules

1 teaspoon honey

Salt and pepper

- Preheat the oven to 210°C/190°C fan (410°F) Gas Mark 6½.

- Using a sharp knife, deeply score the flesh of the butternut halves, without cutting right through. Season with salt and pepper, and drizzle with some olive oil. Place on a baking tray and roast in the oven for 35–40 minutes until tender. During the last few minutes, toast the sourdough in the same oven for 2–3 minutes. Remove from the oven and leave to cool, and increase the oven temperature to 220°C/200°C fan (425°F) Gas Mark 7.

- Meanwhile, cook the macaroni in a pan of boiling salted water for 2 minutes less than the packet suggests, so that it's very al dente.

- Drain and rinse with cold water to halt the cooking, then set aside.

- For the cheese sauce, heat the 1 tablespoon of olive oil in a large pan over a medium heat. Add the flour and cook for 3–5 minutes. Gradually whisk in the milk, adding it a third at a time, until all the milk has been incorporated. Allow the sauce to simmer and thicken, stirring.

- Remove the pan from the heat and stir in the grated cheeses, crumbled stock cube and mustard. Season with salt and pepper to taste.

- For the breadcrumb topping, put the toasted sourdough in a food processor with the parsley, garlic granules and some salt and whizz to crumbs.

- Scoop out the flesh from the butternut and transfer it to a clean blender or food processor.

- Add the béchamel and honey, and blend until silky smooth. Combine the macaroni with the butternut cheese sauce, then pour the mixture into a baking dish or ovenproof skillet.

- Sprinkle the sourdough crumb mixture over the top, then bake in the oven for 6–10 minutes or until the top is golden and bubbling, and the macaroni is fully cooked. Serve hot, ideally with a refreshing side salad.

Prawn and Sriracha Burgers

If you need some new inspiration for burger night, then you have to try my prawn burgers. Quick to prepare, they bring together the zesty citrus hit of lemon, the kick of sriracha and the freshness of prawns, offering a protein-rich meal which won't leave you feeling sluggish.

Makes 2

Time:
30 minutes

Macros:
Under 400kcal,
22g protein per serving

160g (5¾oz) raw peeled prawns (shrimp), roughly chopped

1 spring onion (scallion), roughly chopped

Zest and juice of 1 unwaxed lemon

Handful of parsley leaves

1 tablespoon plain (all-purpose) flour, plus extra for dusting

1 medium free-range egg yolk

1 teaspoon garlic paste

Olive oil, for frying

Salt and pepper

For the salad

1 carrot, peeled

½ cucumber

1 heaped teaspoon peanut butter

Juice of 1 lime

To serve

1 tablespoon sriracha sauce

2 tablespoons thick natural yogurt

2 brioche buns, cut in half

½ medium ripe avocado, sliced

- Add 100g (3½oz) of the prawns to a food processor with the spring onion, lemon zest and juice, parsley, flour, egg yolk, garlic paste and some salt and pepper. Blitz to a coarse mince-like paste; don't over-blend.

- Add the remaining chopped prawns and fold into the mix. Divide the mixture in half and shape into 2 patties, each around 2.5cm (1 inch) thick.

- Use extra flour to lightly coat the outside of the patties, then chill in the refrigerator for at least 20 minutes.

- Meanwhile, use a swivel peeler to pare the carrot and the cucumber into ribbons. Pat dry with kitchen paper and place in a bowl with the peanut butter and lime juice. Using your hands, rub the mixture into the ribbons, then set to one side.

- Mix the sriracha with the yogurt and set aside. Lightly toast the buns.

- Fry the burgers in a little oil in a nonstick frying pan over a medium heat for about 3 minutes on each side, until cooked and golden. Remove from the pan.

- To assemble, spread some sriracha yogurt over the base of the buns, top each with a prawn burger, some sliced avocado and a handful of the dressed vegetables. Replace the bun tops then dive in.

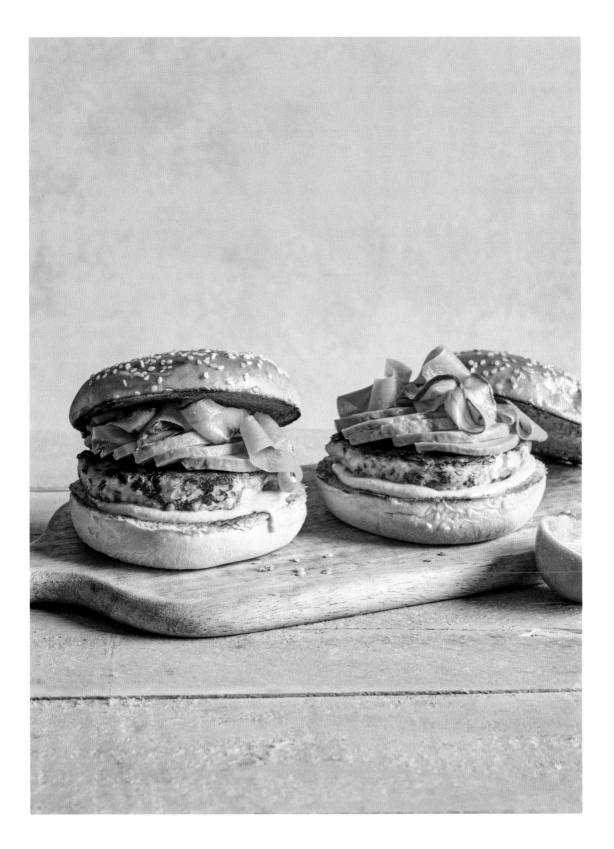

Pesto Prawn Courgetti Linguine

Serves 2

Time:
15 minutes

Macros:
Under 400kcal,
26g protein per serving

Fresh and summery, this recipe was always one of my clients' favourites. The combination of silky linguine, courgette ribbons, sun-dried tomatoes and aromatic basil delivers such a speedy but delicious meal. Rather than cutting out the pasta altogether, I like to combine courgetti and linguine to lighten this up but still keep it super-satisfying.

1 large courgette (zucchini), spiralized using a julienne peeler or pared into ribbons using a swivel peeler

1 teaspoon olive oil

2 banana shallots, diced

2 garlic cloves, minced

2–3 large handfuls of cherry tomatoes

8 sun-dried tomatoes in oil, drained and diced

150g (5½oz) dried linguine

160g (5¾oz) raw peeled prawns (shrimp)

Zest of 1 unwaxed lemon, plus a squeeze of juice

30g (1oz) Parmesan cheese, grated

Generous handful of basil leaves, torn

Salt and pepper

Dried chilli flakes, to serve

- Place the courgette in a colander, sprinkle with a pinch of salt, toss and leave to drain for 5 minutes. Dab dry using kitchen paper, then set aside.

- Heat the olive oil in a deep frying pan over a low-medium heat, then sauté the shallots and garlic with a pinch of salt until translucent. Add the cherry tomatoes and sun-dried tomatoes and continue sautéing for 5 minutes, or until the cherry tomatoes start to burst.

- Meanwhile, cook the linguine in a pan of boiling salted water until al dente. Drain, reserving a cupful of the cooking water.

- Use the back of a wooden spoon to press the tomatoes, releasing their juices. Add 2 tablespoons of the reserved pasta water and the prawns to the pan, allowing the prawns to cook for about 2 minutes. Incorporate the drained pasta, lemon zest, a squeeze of juice, two-thirds of the Parmesan, the basil and a crack of black pepper. Stir well to meld all the flavours, then fold in the courgette ribbons just to warm them through.

- Serve sprinkled with the remaining Parmesan and a pinch of chilli flakes.

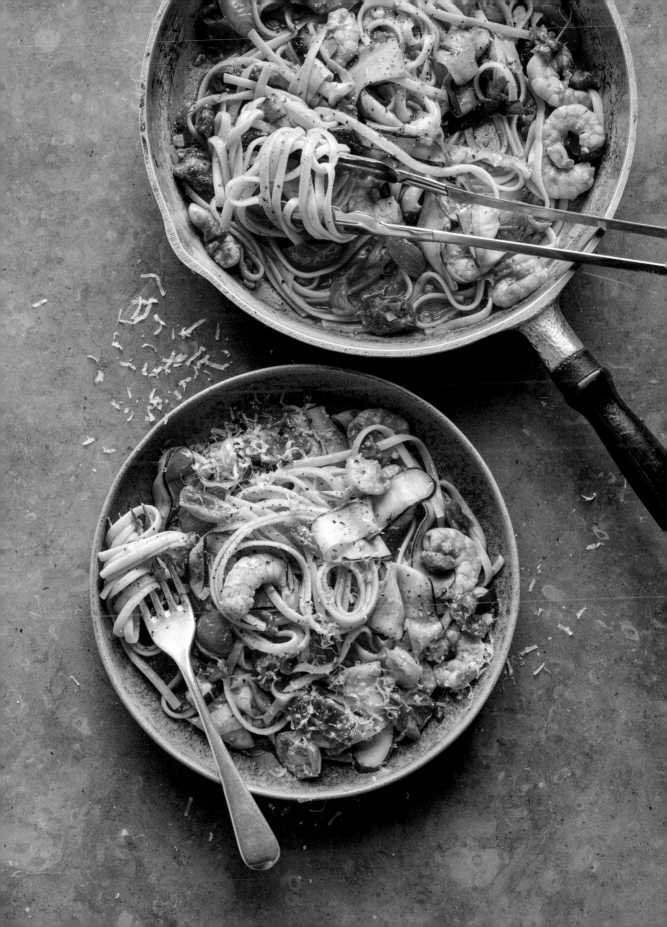

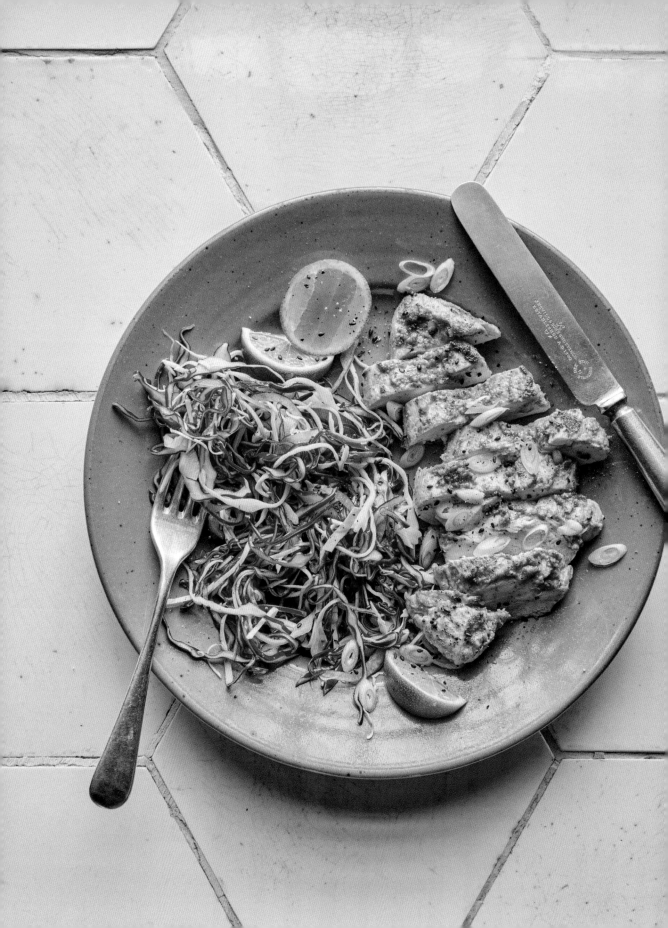

Brick Almond Chicken with Honey and Lime Slaw

Serves 2

Time:
15 minutes,
plus marinating

Macros:
Under 350kcal,
35g protein per serving

The longer you can marinate the chicken, the better it becomes. All the gnarly bits become slightly charred during the cooking process which just gives this dish the most incredible flavour. Almonds are a good source of vitamin E and lots of healthy fats, making them a nutritious addition. Pair with this crisp lime and honey slaw to cut through.

2 boneless, skinless chicken breasts

Olive oil, for cooking

Finely sliced spring onion (scallion), to garnish

For the marinade

1 tablespoon almond butter

2 teaspoons toasted sesame oil

Zest and juice of 1 lime

1 tablespoon light soy sauce

1 garlic clove, minced

1 teaspoon mild curry powder

For the slaw

¼ red cabbage

¼ white cabbage

½ red onion

Zest and juice of 1 lime

1 teaspoon honey

Salt and pepper

- Using a heavy object (like a rolling pin), bash the chicken for about 10 seconds on each side, focusing on the thicker part. You don't want it to become completely flat, just a more even thickness.

- Mix the marinade ingredients together in a deep bowl and rub into the chicken. Cover and place the bowl in the refrigerator for at least an hour, preferably overnight.

- Using a mandolin or swivel peeler, pare both cabbages and the red onion into thin strips and combine in a bowl. Add the lime zest and juice, honey and a pinch each of salt and pepper, and toss to mix. Set aside.

- Heat a frying pan over a medium heat and brush with a bit of olive oil. Pan-fry the marinated chicken breasts for 3–4 minutes on each side, until charred but not burnt. Take off the heat and let them rest in the pan for 2 minutes, then flip and allow them to rest for an additional 3 minutes.

- Serve the slaw alongside the chicken, garnishing the dish with spring onion slices.

My Best Ever Chicken and Tarragon Lasagne

A delightful twist on the classic lasagne, this recipe is perfect for using up the leftover chicken after a roast. The tarragon-spiked béchamel is the star, pulling the whole dish together, but as tarragon isn't always the easiest to find, you can use basil instead, which works well. For the perfect pairing, serve with a balsamic-dressed Italian leaf salad.

Serves 6

Time:
1 hour 15 minutes, plus 15 minutes resting

Macros:
Under 400kcal, 22g protein per serving

---

2 teaspoons olive oil

1 red (bell) pepper, cored, deseeded and diced

1 carrot, diced

1 leek, trimmed, cleaned and diced

1 red onion, diced

1 courgette (zucchini), diced

2 garlic cloves, minced

400g (14oz) cooked chicken leg meat, shredded

10 sun-dried tomatoes in oil, drained and diced

1 heaped teaspoon smoked paprika

Pinch of dried oregano

1 tablespoon tomato purée (paste)

500g (generous 2 cups) passata (puréed canned tomatoes)

1 chicken stock cube, crumbled

2 tablespoons balsamic vinegar

9–12 dried lasagne sheets

Salt and pepper

For the béchamel

2 tablespoons extra virgin olive oil

2 tablespoons plain (all-purpose) flour

800ml (3⅓ cups) semi-skimmed milk

50g (1¾oz) Parmesan cheese, grated, plus extra to assemble

50g (1¾oz) mature Cheddar cheese, grated, plus extra to assemble

1 teaspoon American mustard

Large handful of tarragon, chopped (or use basil)

- Preheat the oven to 220°C/200°C fan (425°F) Gas Mark 7.

- In a large pan, add the olive oil and sauté all the prepared vegetables and garlic, with a pinch of salt and pepper, for 5 minutes over a medium heat.

- Stir in the shredded chicken, the sun-dried tomatoes, smoked paprika, oregano and tomato purée. Continue to cook for another 5 minutes.

- Pour in the passata, then stir in the crumbled stock cube and balsamic vinegar. Allow the mixture to simmer gently for 10–15 minutes.

- Meanwhile, in a separate large pan over a medium heat, combine the olive oil and flour for the béchamel. Cook gently for 3–5 minutes. Gradually whisk in the milk a quarter at a time, until all the milk is used. Allow the sauce to simmer and thicken, stirring.

- Remove from the heat and stir in the grated cheeses, mustard, a generous pinch each of salt and pepper and the chopped tarragon.

- In a 20 x 20cm (8 x 8 inch) ovenproof dish, start the lasagne layering with chicken ragù, followed by some béchamel, a sprinkle of Parmesan, and then a layer of lasagne sheets. Repeat the layers: ragù, béchamel, cheese, pasta, and finish with a thick layer of béchamel. Generously grate some Parmesan and Cheddar over the top, add a light sprinkling of salt and pepper, then bake in the oven for 35 minutes, until golden and bubbling. Allow the lasagne to rest for 15 minutes before serving.

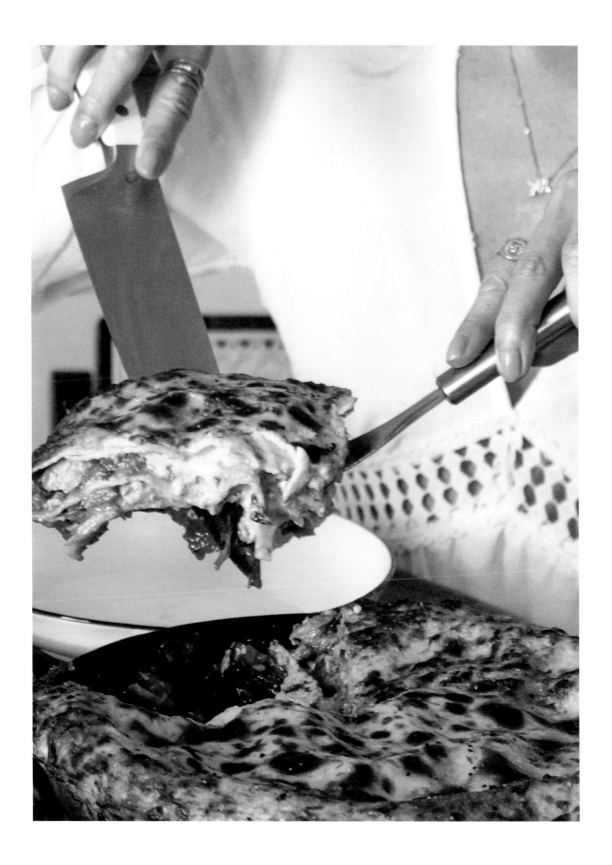

Garlic-crumbed Salmon with Courgettes and Yogurt

Serves 2

Time:
30 minutes

Macros:
Under 600kcal,
50g protein per serving

This dish promises flavours that make you feel like you are in a restaurant. And it's ready in a swift 30 minutes, feeding both your body and mind with every bite. A nutrition-packed seeded garlic crumb paired with omega-3-rich salmon that I have paired with a vibrant sauté of courgettes with protein-packed chickpeas. A true joy to eat!

2 skinless salmon fillets

Dijon mustard, for brushing

1 teaspoon olive oil, plus extra for drizzling

150g (⅔ cup) thick natural yogurt (0% fat)

Juice of ½ lemon

1 teaspoon garlic paste or ½ small garlic clove, crushed

30g (1oz) feta cheese, crumbled

2 spring onions (scallions), diced

400g (14oz) can of chickpeas, drained and rinsed

2 courgettes (zucchini), pared into ribbons using a swivel peeler (avoid the seeded core)

Small handful of basil leaves, roughly torn

15g (½oz) Parmesan cheese, grated

For the crumb

2 slices of seeded bread (about 60g/2¼oz in total)

1 small garlic clove, grated

Small handful of parsley leaves

Zest of 1 unwaxed lemon

15g (½oz) Parmesan cheese, grated

Salt and pepper

- Begin with the crumb. Break the bread into chunks and add to a blender or food processor with the remaining crumb ingredients, and some salt and pepper. Blitz to a fine breadcrumb texture.

- Pat the salmon dry and season with salt. Place on an oven tray, brush a little mustard all over the top and sides of the fillets, then press the breadcrumb mixture onto the fillets. Lightly drizzle with olive oil and refrigerate.

- Preheat the oven to 220°C/200°C fan (425°F) Gas Mark 7 or set an air fryer to 200°C (400°F).

- For the yogurt base, combine the yogurt, lemon juice, garlic and feta in a bowl, mashing the feta into the yogurt for a smooth consistency.

- Transfer the salmon to the oven or air fryer and cook for 8–10 minutes, checking halfway through to ensure the crumb doesn't burn.

- Meanwhile, heat 1 teaspoon of olive oil in a frying pan over a medium heat, then sauté the spring onions and chickpeas for 3–4 minutes. Add the courgette ribbons and basil, cooking for about 2 minutes. Finish with the grated Parmesan, and salt and pepper to taste.

- Plate up the salmon fillets with a base of the yogurt mixture, and the chickpeas and courgette mixture.

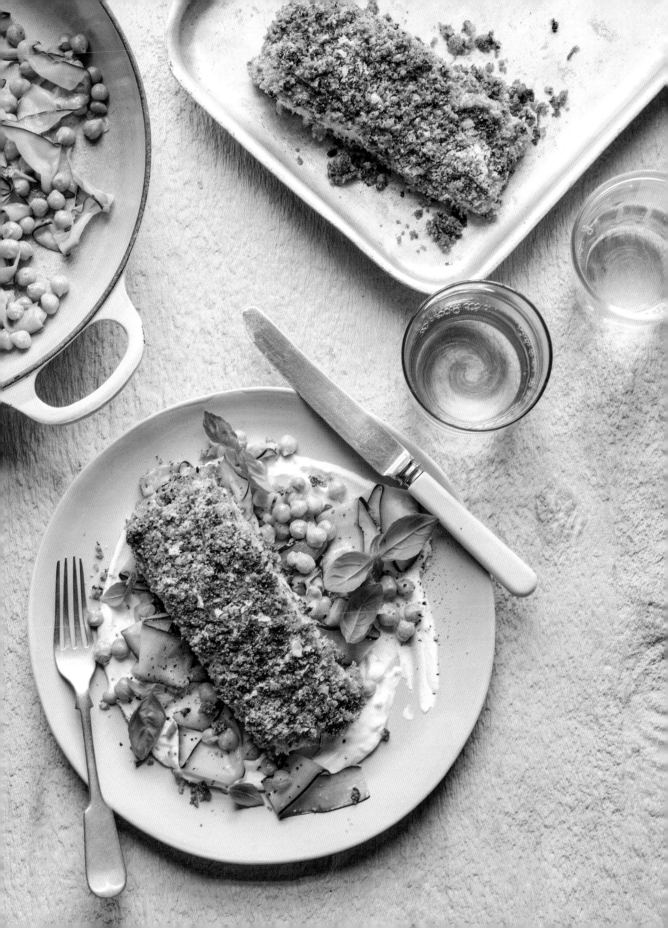

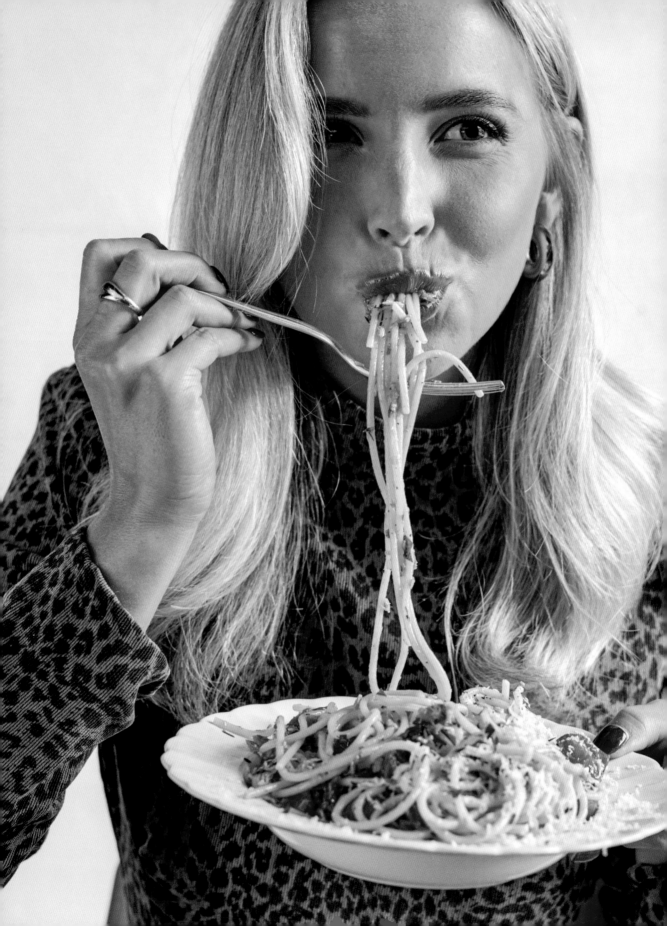

Tuna Puttanesca Spaghetti

Serves 2

Time:
25 minutes

Macros:
Under 350kcal,
28g protein per serving

For those nights when you crave a healthy pasta dish but with minimal effort, this one-dish Tuna Puttanesca Spaghetti does not disappoint. Don't be fooled by its simplicity, this dish is packed with so much flavour and contains mostly store-cupboard ingredients too, so it's often the perfect thing to throw together if your refrigerator is looking a little sparse.

250g (9oz) cherry tomatoes

12 pitted Kalamata olives, halved

1 tablespoon capers

2 large garlic cloves, finely chopped

4 anchovies in oil, drained and roughly chopped

½ teaspoon dried oregano

½ small red chilli, deseeded (if desired) and diced

Generous drizzle of extra virgin olive oil

150g (5½oz) dried spaghetti

120g (4¼oz) drained canned tuna

Small handful of parsley, chopped

20g (¾oz) Parmesan cheese, grated, plus extra to serve

Squeeze of lemon juice

Salt and pepper

- Preheat the oven to 220°C/200°C fan (425°F) Gas Mark 7.

- In a deep baking dish, combine the cherry tomatoes, olives, capers, garlic, anchovies, oregano and chilli. Season with salt and pepper and drizzle over the extra virgin olive oil. Stir to mix, then transfer to the oven and bake for 15 minutes.

- Meanwhile, cook the spaghetti in a pan of boiling salted water until al dente. Drain, reserving a cupful of the pasta cooking water.

- Remove the dish from the oven, gently press down on the tomatoes to release their juices, add the tuna and mix into the sauce.

- Toss through the parsley, Parmesan, a little squeeze of lemon juice and the drained spaghetti. If the mixture seems dry, add a splash of the reserved pasta water and toss until unctuous.

- Serve with an extra flurry of Parmesan.

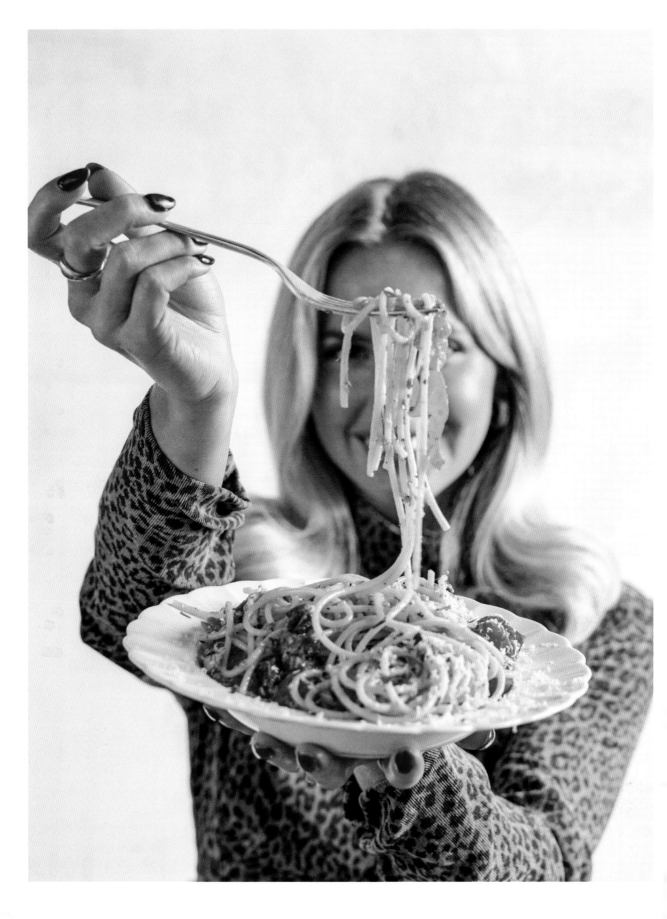

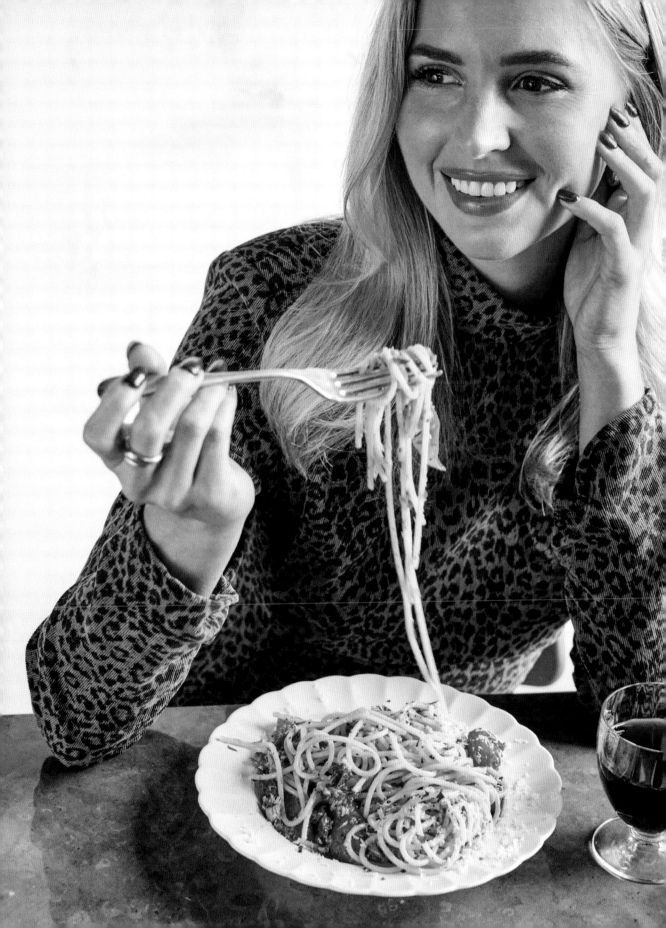

Chicken and Greens Pot Pie

This recipe is the perfect example of how foods we are made to believe are 'bad' for us can be balanced, nourishing and part of any healthy diet. This pie is filled to the brim with nutrient-rich greens, fresh thyme and roasted chicken. Top with a layer of flaky puff pastry and bake. This is one of my favourite recipes to use up leftover chicken you may have from a Sunday roast.

Serves 4

Time:
30 minutes (plus 30 minutes baking time)

Macros:
Under 400kcal,
47g protein per serving

1 tablespoon olive oil

1 leek, trimmed, cleaned and diced

1 shallot or small white onion, diced

1 courgette (zucchini), diced

2 garlic cloves, finely diced

Few sprigs of thyme, leaves stripped

1 heaped tablespoon plain (all-purpose) flour

250ml (generous 1 cup) semi-skimmed milk

1 chicken stock cube, crumbled

Handful of chopped kale, spinach or cavolo nero

300g (10½oz) roasted chicken meat, roughly chopped

100g (⅔ cup) frozen peas

1 heaped teaspoon wholegrain mustard

Zest of ½ unwaxed lemon, plus a squeeze of juice

20g (¾oz) Parmesan cheese, grated

1 tablespoon half-fat crème fraîche

320g (11¼oz) sheet of ready-rolled puff pastry

1 medium free-range egg, beaten, to glaze

Salt and pepper

- Heat the oil in a large pan over a medium heat and add the leek, shallot or onion, courgette and garlic, the thyme and a pinch each of salt and pepper. Sauté for about 10 minutes to soften.

- Stir in the flour and let it cook for a few moments. Mix in a splash of water to form a smooth paste, then add the milk and the stock cube. Allow the mixture to simmer and thicken for about 5 minutes. Next, add the chopped greens, roasted chicken, frozen peas and mustard.

- Let it simmer briefly before stirring through the lemon zest, a squeeze of lemon juice, the Parmesan, crème fraîche, and additional seasoning if required.

- Transfer the mixture to a pie dish or another ovenproof dish and let it cool for 5 minutes.

- Meanwhile, preheat the oven to 200°C/180°C fan (400°F) Gas Mark 6.

- Drape the puff pastry over the pie/ovenproof dish, trimming any overhang. Crimp the edges, cut 4 small vents in the centre, and brush with the beaten egg. Finish with a pinch of salt and a crack of black pepper on top.

- Bake in the oven for 30 minutes or until the pastry is puffed up and golden-brown.

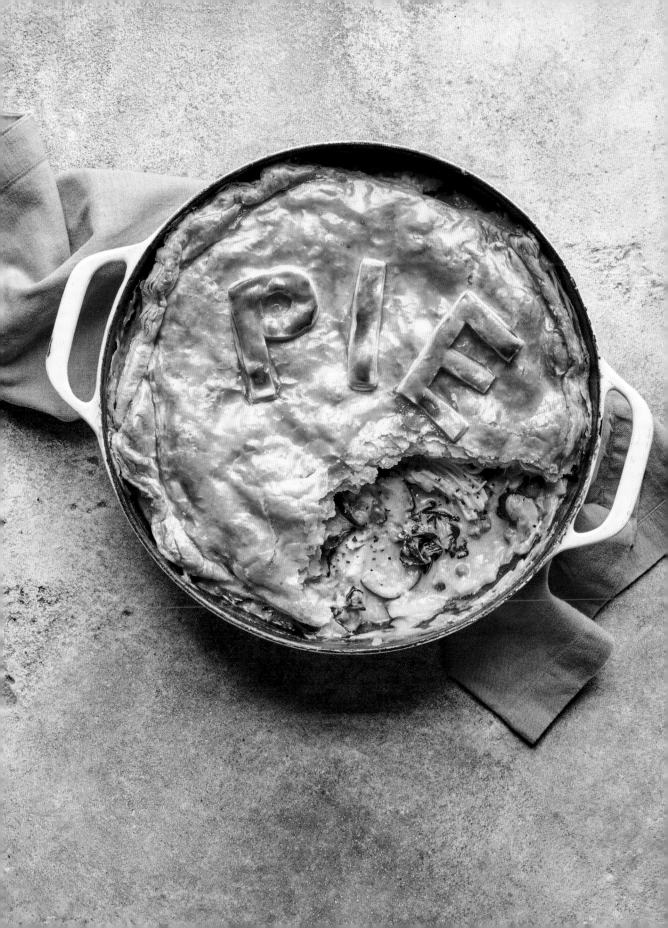

'Ratatouille' Orzo with Sea Bass

Some recipes just taste like sunshine and this is certainly one of them. My favourite way to prepare orzo, inspired by the flavour of ratatouille but paired with a bright sun-dried tomato dressing that just tastes like summer. The diversity of vegetables adds essential vitamins and fibre, vitamin C and antioxidants. This recipe is a reliable choice for dinner parties and works well as a barbecue side dish, no matter the weather.

Serves 4

Time:
35 minutes

Macros:
Under 450kcal,
28g protein per serving

---

4 sea bass fillets

For the orzo base

1 courgette (zucchini)

1 red (bell) pepper, cored and deseeded

1 yellow (bell) pepper, cored and deseeded

1 teaspoon olive oil, plus extra for the sea bass pan

1 teaspoon dried oregano

½ teaspoon garlic granules

Handful of basil leaves, chopped

200g (7oz) dried orzo

80g (2¾oz) feta cheese, crumbled

1 red onion, very finely chopped

Handful of pitted Kalamata olives, roughly chopped

150g (5½oz) cherry tomatoes, halved

Salt and pepper

For the dressing

1 tablespoon extra virgin olive oil

Juice of 1 lemon

1 tablespoon sun-dried tomato paste

1 teaspoon Dijon mustard

2 teaspoons honey

- Preheat the oven to 220°C/200°C fan (425°F) Gas Mark 7.

- Dice your courgette and peppers in similar-sized pieces, and toss in the olive oil, oregano, garlic granules and some salt and pepper. Tip onto a baking tray in a single layer and roast in the oven for 20–25 minutes until golden. Remove from the oven and toss through the basil.

- While the vegetables are roasting, cook the orzo in a pan of boiling salted water according to the packet instructions, then drain, rinse under cold water to remove the starch to stop it sticking, and set aside.

- Make the dressing by whisking the olive oil, lemon juice, sun-dried tomato paste, Dijon mustard and honey together in a small bowl, with salt and pepper to taste.

- Mix the cooked orzo with the roasted vegetables, crumbled feta, red onion, olives and tomatoes. Add half the dressing and mix through.

- Dry the sea bass fillets and season with salt. Cook the sea bass fillets, skin-side down, over a medium heat in a oiled frying pan for 3 minutes, so the skin crisps, then flip them over and remove the pan from the heat. Remove the cooked fillets from the pan after 30 seconds.

- For each serving, portion the orzo with a sea bass fillet, add an extra drizzle of dressing and dive in.

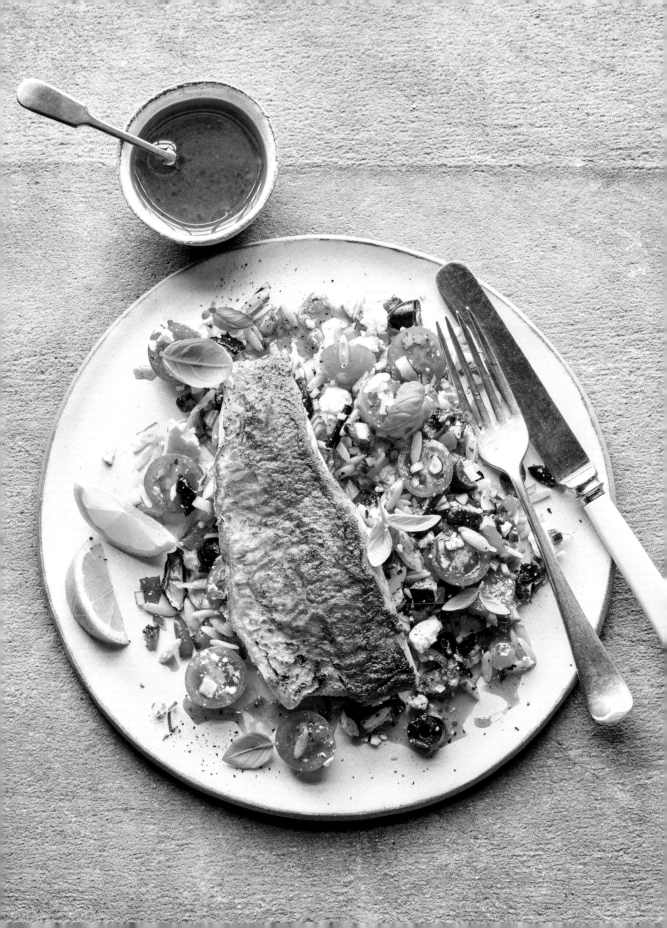

Sticky Peanut Stir Fry

This Sticky Peanut Stir Fry is one of my go-to meals when I want something quick and delicious and that uses ingredients that I always have in my cupboard. I like to pair this with rice but it's equally delicious with noodles. Makes fantastic leftovers too. Feel free to use whatever vegetables you need to use up in your refrigerator, and swap the protein to suit you. Have your chicken and veg prepped prior to starting: the actual cooking process here is super speedy.

Serves 2

Time:
20 minutes

Macros:
Under 500kcal,
30g protein per serving

100g (½ cup) brown rice

2 teaspoons neutral-flavoured oil

300g (10½oz) boneless, skinless chicken breast, cut into thin strips (or use tofu, raw peeled prawns (shrimp) or raw beef)

1 tablespoon light soy sauce

3 spring onions (scallions), sliced into chunks, plus extra thin slices to serve

½ red chilli, deseeded and finely diced

1 garlic clove, minced

1 carrot, cut into matchsticks

1 red (bell) pepper, cored, deseeded and cut into thin strips

150g (5½oz) Tenderstem broccoli, each stem cut into 3

2 tablespoons roasted salted peanuts

Salt

For the stir-fry sauce

1 tablespoon peanut butter

2 tablespoons light soy sauce

1 teaspoon rice vinegar

Zest and juice of ½ lime

1 garlic clove, minced

1 heaped teaspoon honey

- Cook your rice in a pan of boiling salted water, according to the packet instructions, then drain.

- Meanwhile, make the stir-fry sauce by mixing the peanut butter, soy sauce, rice vinegar, lime zest and juice, garlic and honey together in a small bowl until smooth. Set aside.

- Heat a nonstick frying pan or wok over a high heat, add 1 teaspoon of the oil, then add the chicken strips and soy sauce. Stir-fry for 3–4 minutes until browned, then remove to a plate.

- Add the remaining teaspoon of oil to the same pan, then stir-fry the spring onions, chilli and garlic, moving them around the pan constantly so they don't catch. Add the carrot, red pepper and broccoli and stir-fry for 3 minutes, then add the chicken strips back in with the roasted peanuts and the sauce.

- Cook until sticky, caramelised and bubbling. Finish with a scattering of extra spring onion slices and serve with the cooked rice.

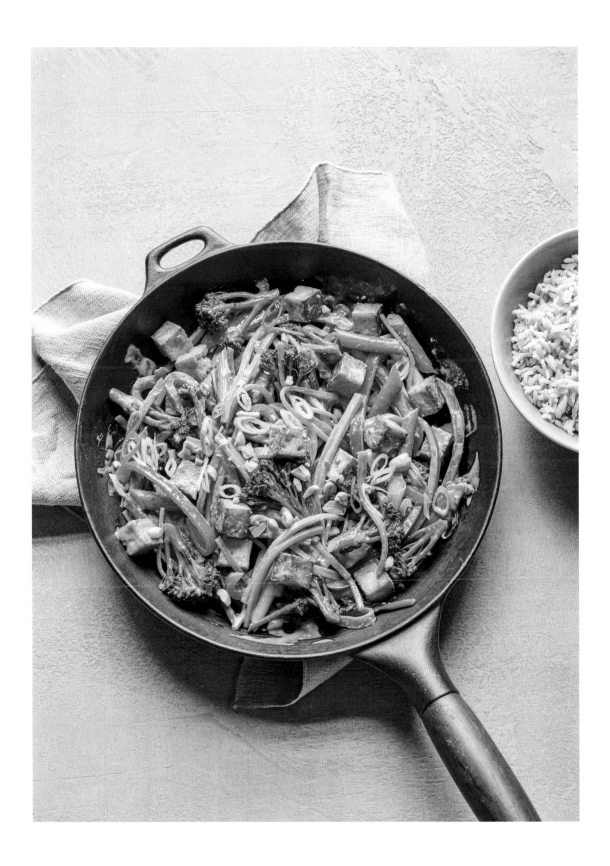

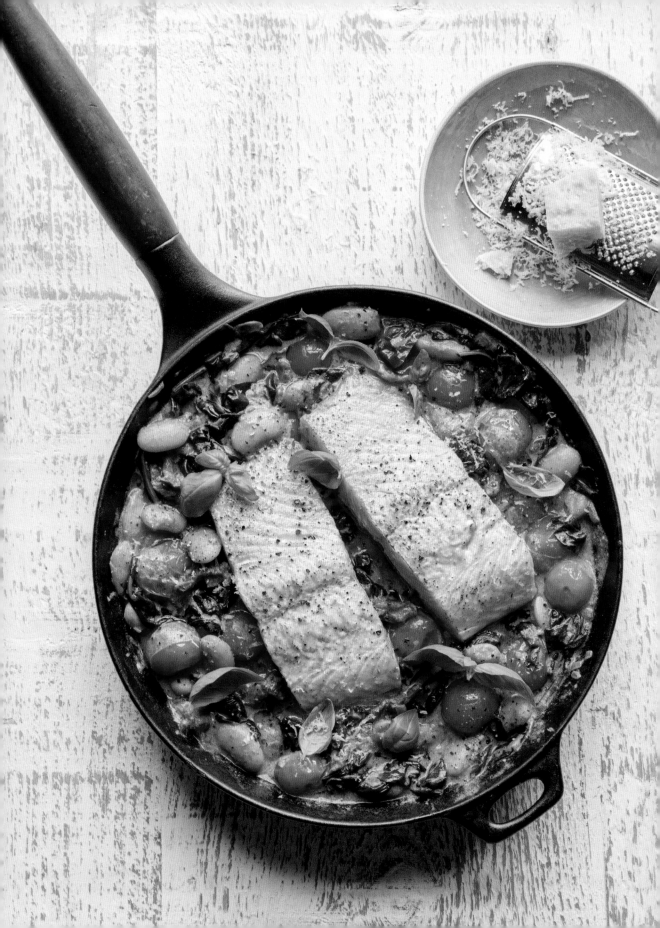

One-pan Tuscan Salmon

This viral hit is one of the most popular recipes on my social channels. An easy all-in-one-pan meal, this is perfect for simple but delicious midweek dinners. Ready in just 25 minutes, it's creamy but still has a light freshness. Butter beans provide a source of complex carbohydrates, protein and fibre to make this perfectly filling.

Serves 2

Time:
25 minutes

Macros:
Under 500kcal,
38g protein per serving

2 skinless salmon fillets

1 teaspoon olive oil

1 shallot, diced

2 garlic cloves, minced

200g (7oz) cherry tomatoes

8 sun-dried tomatoes in oil, drained and chopped

½ teaspoon smoked paprika

Small handful of basil, stems and leaves separated and chopped, plus extra leaves to serve

1 chicken stock cube, crumbled

200ml (scant 1 cup) water

400g (14oz) can of butter beans (lima beans), drained and rinsed

2 tablespoons half-fat crème fraîche

Zest of ½ unwaxed lemon

15g (½oz) Parmesan cheese, grated, plus extra for serving

Few handfuls of baby spinach leaves

Salt and pepper

- Season the salmon fillets with salt and pepper. Heat a frying pan until hot, then add the salmon and sear on all sides until coloured. Remove and set to one side.

- In the same pan, reduce the heat a little, add the olive oil, then sweat the shallot and garlic with a pinch of salt for 5 minutes. Add the whole cherry tomatoes, sun-dried tomatoes, smoked paprika and chopped basil stems.

- Sauté for a few minutes, then add the stock cube and the water. Bring to a simmer, then add the butter beans and let it simmer for another 5 minutes.

- Reduce the heat to low, then mix in the crème fraîche, lemon zest, Parmesan and a crack of black pepper. Stir in the spinach and chopped basil leaves.

- Position the salmon fillets in the pan and allow them to warm and cook through.

- Serve sprinkled with extra basil leaves and a grating of Parmesan.

Meatball and Ricotta Al Forno

Serves 4

Time:
55 minutes

Macros:
Under 550kcal,
50g protein per serving

Meatballs have always been a classic dinner staple for me and this is one of my favourite flavour combinations – soft ricotta-spiked meatballs made with lean minced beef paired with a sun-dried tomato ragù. I have added nutrient-dense butter beans for a balanced source of carbohydrates and additional plant protein. Store leftovers in the refrigerator for 3 days.

500g (1lb 2oz) 5% fat minced (ground) beef

2 heaped tablespoons ricotta cheese

Zest of 1 unwaxed lemon

80g (2¾oz) fresh wholemeal (wholewheat) bread-crumbs (made from blitzed stale bread)

30g (1oz) Parmesan cheese, grated

1 medium free-range egg

Large handful of basil, leaves chopped (save the stems for the sauce), plus extra to garnish

1 tablespoon olive oil

Salt and pepper

For the sauce

1 medium courgette (zucchini), diced

1 red (bell) pepper, cored, deseeded and diced

1 red onion, diced

1 garlic clove, minced

1 tablespoon sun-dried tomato paste

1 tablespoon tomato purée (paste)

Small handful of chopped basil stems

400g (14oz) can of butter beans (lima beans), drained and rinsed

1 teaspoon smoked paprika

500g (generous 2 cups) passata (puréed canned tomatoes)

1 chicken stock cube, crumbled

2 tablespoons balsamic vinegar

To finish

20g (¾oz) Parmesan cheese, grated

5–6 tablespoons ricotta cheese

- Preheat the oven to 220°C/200°C fan (425°F) Gas Mark 7.

- In a bowl, prepare the meatballs. Combine the minced beef, ricotta, lemon zest, breadcrumbs, Parmesan, egg and chopped basil leaves. Season with salt and pepper. The mix should feel slightly wet. Take care not to over-mix, as this can result in tough meatballs. Form the mixture into medium-sized balls (about 5cm/2 inches), using your hands.

- Heat the oil in a large ovenproof pan or flameproof casserole over a medium heat and, in batches, brown the meatballs on all sides. They should be coloured but not cooked through. Remove them as they brown from the pan, and set aside.

- In the same pan, for the sauce, add the diced vegetables and garlic with a pinch of salt, and sauté over a medium heat for 5 minutes. Stir in the sun-dried tomato paste and tomato purée along with the chopped basil stems, and cook for another 5 minutes.

- Add the butter beans, smoked paprika, passata and stock cube. Half-fill the passata container with water and add this to the pan. Simmer for 10 minutes until thickened. Finish with the balsamic vinegar and adjust the seasoning to taste.

- Place the meatballs in the sauce, sprinkle over the Parmesan, and dot the ricotta on top.

- Bake in the oven for 15–20 minutes, until the sauce is thick and rich, and the meatballs are cooked through. Garnish with basil leaves.

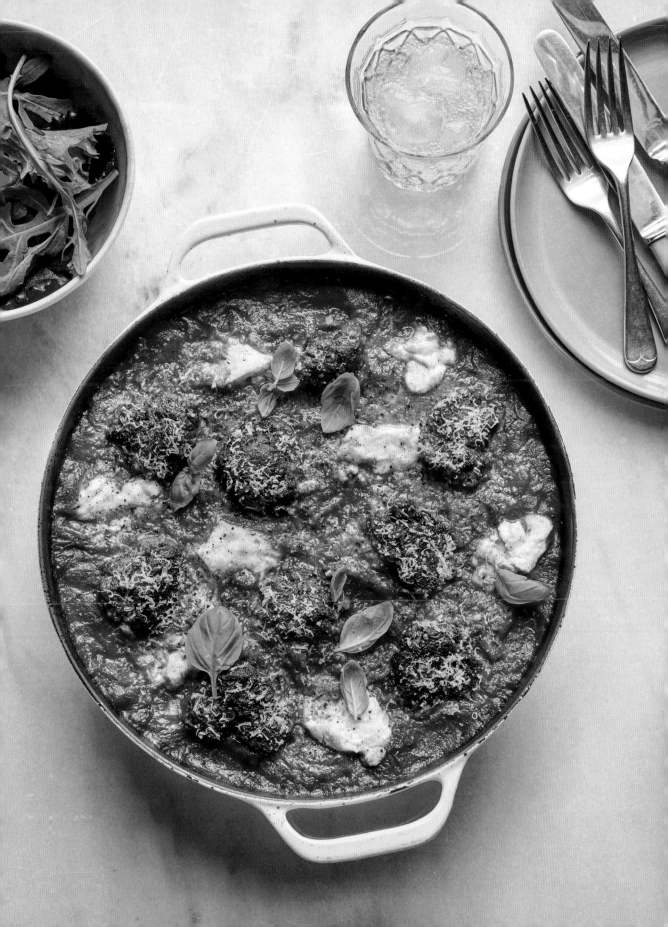

Smoky Mexican Black Bean Soup

Serves 2

Time:
30 minutes

Macros:
Under 350kcal, 18g
protein per serving

A fiery and fresh soup inspired by a Mexican burrito. Black beans are an excellent plant-based source of protein and fibre. Finish with all the classic toppings for the ultimate midweek meal.

2 teaspoons olive oil

1 red onion, finely chopped

1 red (bell) pepper, cored, deseeded and cut into chunks

2 garlic cloves, chopped

1 teaspoon chilli powder

1 teaspoon ground coriander

1 teaspoon smoked paprika

1 tablespoon sun-dried tomato paste

400g (14oz) can of chopped tomatoes

400g (14oz) can of black beans, drained and rinsed

1 chicken stock cube, crumbled and dissolved in 300ml (1¼ cups) boiling water

Salt and pepper

To serve
½ ripe avocado, peeled, stoned and diced

15g (½oz) feta cheese, crumbled

Small handful of coriander (cilantro) leaves, chopped

Soured cream

1 lime, cut into wedges

- Heat the oil in a medium pan over a medium heat. Add the red onion and pepper and sweat, stirring occasionally, for about 10 minutes, until they soften and the onion becomes translucent.

- Stir in the garlic, chilli powder, ground coriander, smoked paprika and sun-dried tomato paste. Mix and sauté for a few extra minutes.

- Tip in the canned tomatoes, black beans and chicken stock. Stir everything together, ensuring the ingredients are well incorporated.

- Cover the pan and let the soup simmer for about 15 minutes, then season to taste.

- Meanwhile, prepare the toppings.

- Once the soup is ready, ladle it into bowls and top each portion with some of the avocado, feta and coriander, and a dollop of soured cream. Place a lime wedge on the side for added zing.

Fish Pie with Garlic and Parmesan Crumb

I adore fish pie, it's one of my favourite classic dishes. A creamy fish pie filling packed with goodness with the most delicious garlic and Parmesan crumb. You can assemble this in individual portions and freeze them for ease – simply thaw overnight and then bake in the oven until piping hot, golden and bubbling.

Serves 4

Time:
1 hour

Macros:
Under 500kcal, 40g protein per serving

For the mash

1kg (2lb 4oz) white potatoes, peeled and cut into chunks

Splash of semi-skimmed milk

1 tablespoon extra virgin olive oil

For the filling

2 teaspoons olive oil

2 banana shallots, diced

2 garlic cloves, minced

1 leek, trimmed, cleaned and finely diced

1 courgette (zucchini), finely diced

1 tablespoon plain (all-purpose) flour

400ml (1⅔ cups) semi-skimmed milk

1 chicken stock cube, crumbled

1 tablespoon American mustard

2 handfuls of baby spinach leaves

Zest of 1 unwaxed lemon

300g (10½oz) fish pie mix (salmon, smoked haddock, etc.)

160g (5¾oz) raw peeled prawns (shrimp)

Salt and pepper

For the crumb

80g (2¾oz) granary bread

Handful of parsley leaves

Zest of ½ unwaxed lemon

20g (¾oz) Parmesan cheese, grated

1 teaspoon garlic granules

- Preheat the oven to 220°C/200°C fan (425°F) Gas Mark 7.

- Put the potatoes in a large pan, cover with water, bring to the boil and cook for 10–15 minutes until cooked through. Drain thoroughly, return to the pan and add the splash of milk and the extra virgin olive oil. Mash together well, seasoning with salt and pepper.

- Heat a separate large pan over a medium heat, add the olive oil and sweat the shallots, garlic, leek and courgette with a pinch of salt for 5 minutes until softened.

- Stir in the flour, then whisk in the milk until smooth. Add the stock cube, mustard, spinach leaves and lemon zest and simmer gently until slightly thickened. Season with a pinch each of salt and pepper. Fold the fish pie mix and prawns evenly through the sauce, take off the heat and then tip into an ovenproof baking dish and allow to cool slightly.

- In a food processor, blitz all the crumb ingredients together to form a rough crumb.

- Top the fish pie mixture with the mashed potato. Scatter over the crumb and bake in the oven for 15–20 minutes until bubbling, taking care that the crumb doesn't burn. Leave to rest out of the oven for 5 minutes before serving.

Salmon and Sexy Veg

Serves 2

Time:
15 minutes

Macros:
Under 350kcal,
22g protein per serving

I see people turn to 'protein and veg'-based meals so often when they embark on a 'health kick'. The most crucial aspect for me is that meals always have to taste delicious, even if they are part of a conscious effort to eat healthily. This is my take on protein and vegetables: simple, adaptable, and ready in under 15 minutes. I eat this nearly every week!

2 salmon fillets, skin on
4 anchovies in oil, drained and roughly chopped
½ red chilli, deseeded and finely diced
2 garlic cloves, roughly chopped
1 tablespoon capers, roughly chopped
Zest and juice of 1 unwaxed lemon
2 teaspoons extra virgin olive oil, plus extra for frying
350g (12oz) Tenderstem broccoli
1 tablespoon water
Salt and pepper

- Dry the salmon fillets well and season them with salt and pepper. Place them, skin-side up, in the refrigerator while you prepare your flavour base.

- In a pestle and mortar, combine the anchovies, chilli, garlic, capers and lemon zest and juice. Add the extra virgin olive oil and mash everything together to form a rough paste. Season with a pinch of salt and set aside.

- Heat a frying pan over a medium-high heat, with a little olive oil added. Place the salmon, skin-side down in the pan, pressing gently to seal. Let it cook for 4 minutes, so the skin crisps.

- Meanwhile, heat a second frying pan over a medium-high heat and add a dash of olive oil and the broccoli. Allow it to blister slightly for 2 minutes, then pour in the water to steam the broccoli. Once the water has evaporated, add the paste you prepared earlier and sauté for a few minutes while you finish cooking the salmon.

- Flip the salmon and sear the other side for 2 minutes, then remove from the pan.

- To serve, dish up a crispy-skin salmon fillet alongside the sautéed broccoli. Pair with a grain such as quinoa or rice, if needed.

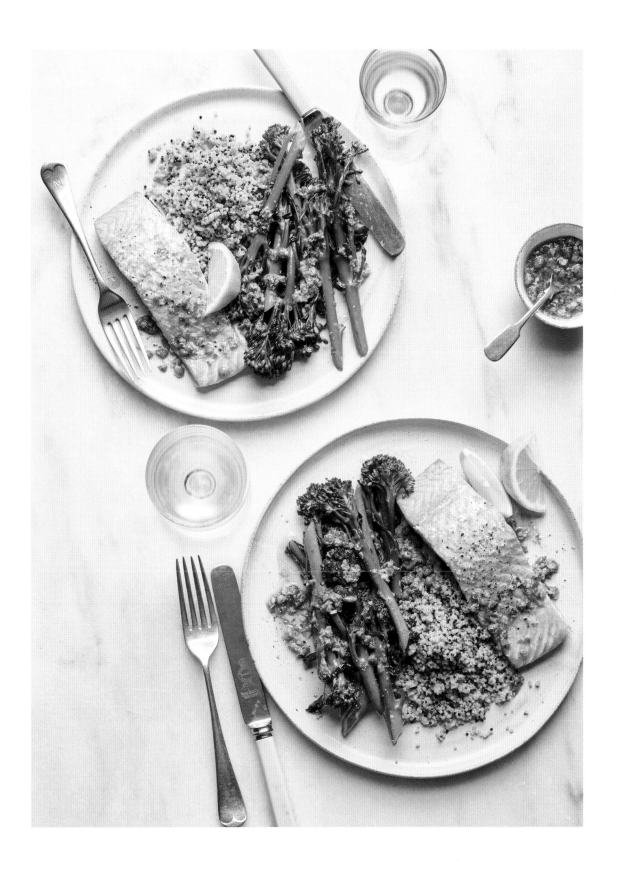

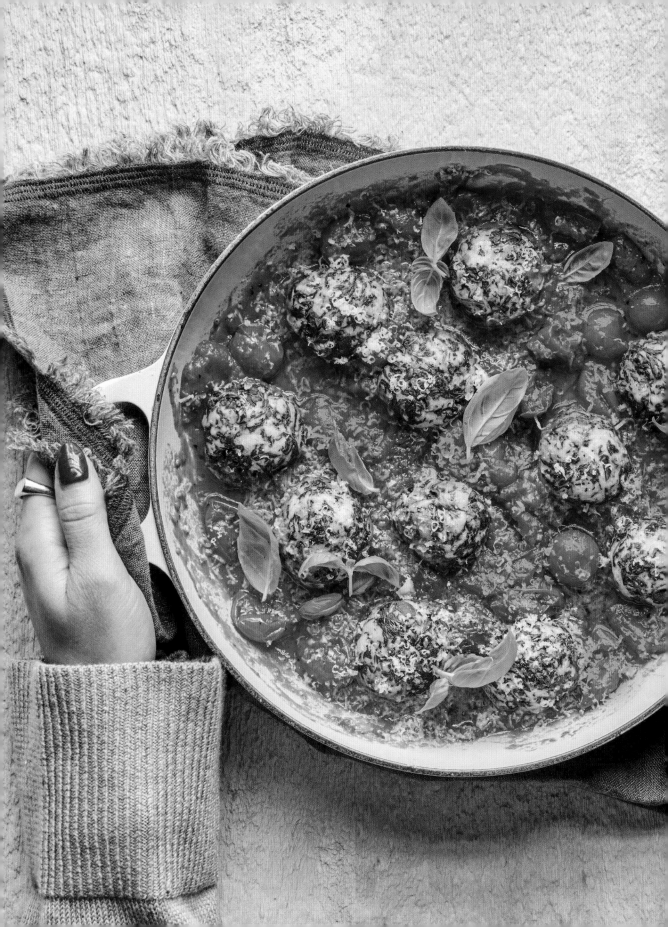

Spinach and Ricotta Malfatti

Though vaguely resembling a giant gnocchi, malfatti are made from a simple mixture of ricotta, Parmesan, egg and spinach. The result is a gorgeous, light and fluffy dumpling. Ricotta is a great source of selenium, an important antioxidant mineral which plays a role in protecting the body from free radical damage and oxidative stress. Paired with nutrient-dense spinach and tomatoes and full of complete protein, it will keep you fuelled for longer.

Serves 2

Time:
30 minutes

Macros:
Under 400kcal,
20g protein per serving

250g (9oz) spinach leaves

125g (generous ½ cup) ricotta cheese

1 medium free-range egg yolk

30g (4 tablespoons) plain (all-purpose) flour, plus extra for dusting

60g (2¼oz) Parmesan cheese, grated, plus extra to serve

Zest of 1 unwaxed lemon

Salt and pepper

For the tomato sauce

1 tablespoon olive oil

1 teaspoon chopped garlic

1 red chilli, deseeded and finely diced

30g (1oz) basil, stems chopped and leaves torn (keep separate)

400g (14oz) can of cherry tomatoes

- Rinse the spinach and put into a saucepan. Place over a medium heat and cook, covered, for a few minutes, until wilted. Tip into a sieve (strainer) and leave until cool enough to handle, then squeeze out as much water as possible. Transfer the drained spinach to a chopping board and finely chop.

- In a mixing bowl, combine the ricotta, egg yolk, flour, Parmesan, lemon zest and chopped spinach. Mix thoroughly, seasoning generously with salt and pepper.

- On a well-floured board, gently roll the mixture into 4cm (1½ inch) balls. As the mixture can be wet, handle it delicately and use the flour to prevent sticking.

- For the tomato sauce, heat the olive oil in a deep saucepan or sauté pan, then sauté the garlic, chilli and chopped basil stems for a few minutes. Add the canned cherry tomatoes, season with salt and pepper and let it simmer for 5 minutes, gently pressing the tomatoes with the back of a wooden spoon so they slightly burst. Add the torn basil leaves and stir.

- One at a time, gently place each malfatti in the tomato sauce. Cover with a lid to allow the malfatti to steam, and cook for about 5 minutes, or until the malfatti expand slightly and the sauce reduces.

- Let it cool for a few minutes before serving, generously topped with grated Parmesan.

Creamy Coconut Thai Green Noodles

Who doesn't love a big bowl of comforting noodles? I am always surprised by how quick this meal is to make for the amount of flavour it delivers. A silky coconut broth is bright, vibrant and full of aromatic goodness, perfect for slurping. Swap the salmon for any protein of choice.

Serves 2

Time:
30 minutes

Macros:
Under 600kcal,
35g protein per serving

2 skinless salmon fillets

½ teaspoon garlic granules

Pinch of dried chilli flakes

1 heaped tablespoon Thai green curry paste

2 large spring onions (scallion), chopped

1 red (bell) pepper, cored, deseeded and cut into strips

100g (3½oz) Tenderstem broccoli, cut into chunks

1 carrot, julienned

400g (14oz) can of light coconut milk

½ chicken stock cube, crumbled

Zest of 1 lime and juice of ½

1 teaspoon honey

1 tablespoon light soy sauce

1 tablespoon fish sauce

2 nests of dried egg noodles

Salt

To garnish

Small handful of coriander (cilantro) leaves

Chopped spring onion (scallion)

Crispy chilli oil (optional)

- Preheat the oven to 220°C/200°C fan (425°F) Gas Mark 7 or set an air fryer to 200°C (400°F).

- Season the salmon fillets with some salt, the garlic granules and chilli flakes. Place on an oven tray and cook in the oven for 12 minutes or in the air fryer for 8 minutes, until fully cooked.

- As the salmon cooks, warm the curry paste over a medium heat in a deep pan until it begins to sizzle. Stir in the spring onions, red pepper, broccoli and carrot.

- Add the coconut milk to the pan, refill the can with water and add that too, then bring to a gentle simmer. Add the chicken stock cube with the lime zest and juice, honey, soy sauce and fish sauce.

- Add the noodles and simmer until the noodles are tender but the vegetables still have a little bite. Taste and add more lime juice, soy or fish sauce as desired.

- To serve, ladle the noodles and sauce into bowls. Garnish with coriander and spring onion. Place a cooked salmon fillet on top and, if desired, drizzle with crispy chilli oil.

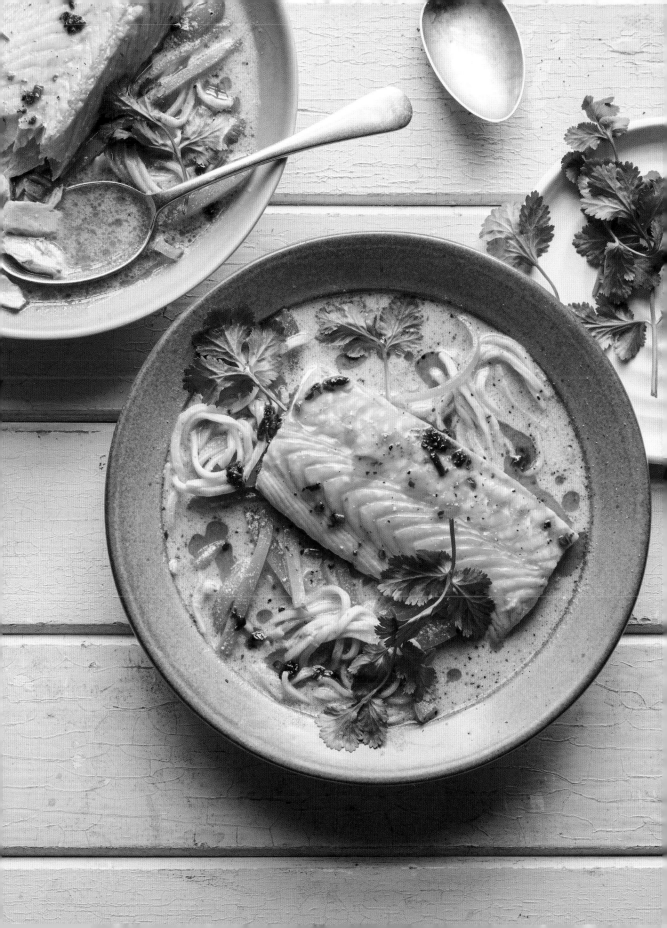

Superfood Vegetarian Bolognese

Serves 6

Time:
1 hour

Macros:
Under 200kcal,
7g protein per serving

My Superfood Vegetarian Bolognese gets its title because it's packed full of eight different plant varieties. It's perfect for batch cooking, freezing and using for a variety of meals. Pair with pasta, bake into a cottage pie and even stuff into a jacket potato. There is a little effort involved in chopping (use a food processor for ease, if you like), but it's so rewarding – good enough to please any meat eater!

1 tablespoon olive oil

1 white onion, finely diced

1 leek, trimmed, cleaned and finely chopped

2 celery sticks, finely diced

2 carrots, peeled and finely diced

Sprig of rosemary, leaves stripped

1 courgette (zucchini), finely diced

2–3 handfuls of mushrooms, finely diced

175ml (¾ cup) red wine

500g (1lb 2oz) cooked green lentils
(from a can or pouch)

500g (generous 2 cups) passata
(puréed canned tomatoes)

400g (14oz) can of chopped tomatoes

1 tablespoon tomato purée (paste)

1 tablespoon sun-dried tomato paste

1 vegetable stock cube, crumbled

2 tablespoons balsamic vinegar

30g (1oz) basil leaves

Salt and pepper

- Heat the olive oil in a pan over a medium heat, add the onion, leek, celery, carrots and rosemary, with a pinch of salt, and sweat for 5 minutes. Add the courgette and mushrooms and continue to sweat for another 10–15 minutes, or until starting to colour and turn golden.

- Pour in the wine and reduce down over a high heat for 3 minutes. Add the lentils, passata, canned tomatoes, tomato purée and sun-dried tomato paste. Half-fill the chopped tomato can with water and add the stock cube, then tip into the pot and season with pepper and the balsamic vinegar.

- Let the mixture simmer, uncovered, over a medium heat for 25–30 minutes, or until thickened and reduced. Taste and season again if needed, then tear in the basil leaves and serve with pasta, as a cottage pie or in a jacket potato.

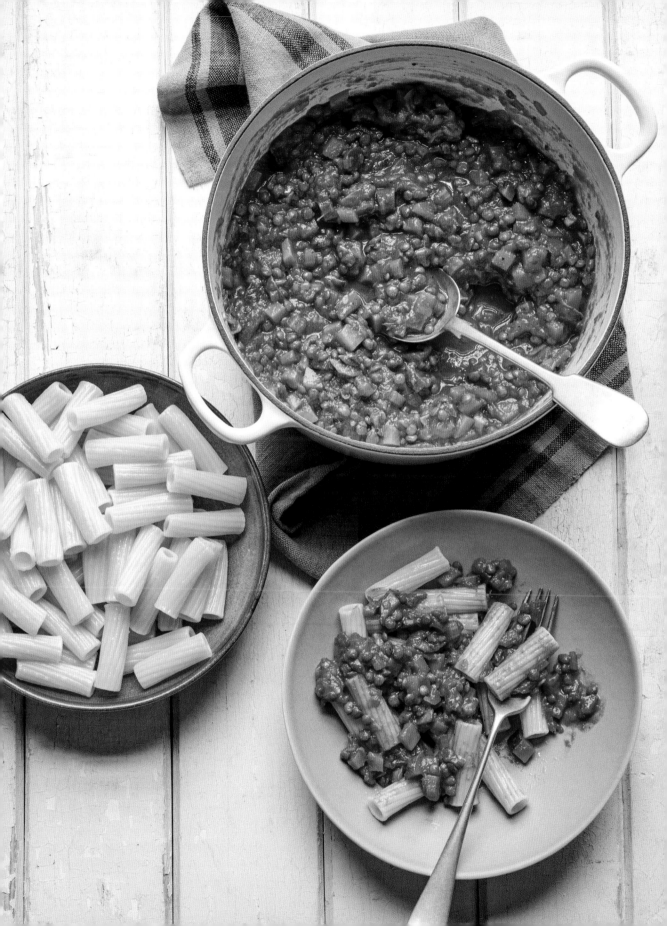

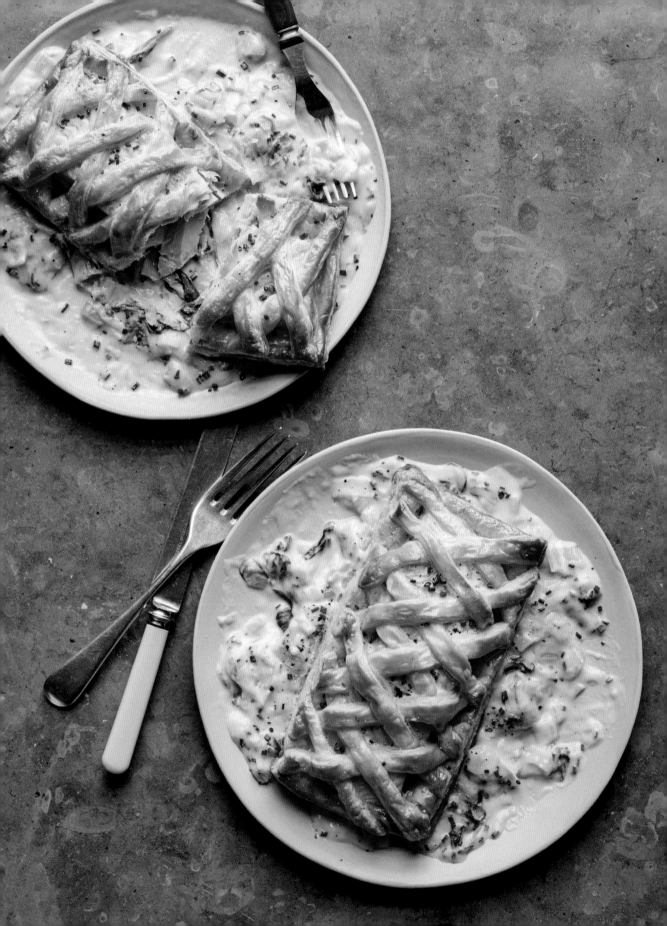

Individual Salmon en Croûte

This dish holds a special place in my heart. Growing up, I would always request it from my mum for special occasions, or when I just needed cheering up. In our household, we simply call it 'salmon in puff' – buttery, omega-3-rich salmon enveloped in a puff pastry lattice, served alongside sautéed leeks. I hope it brings as much joy to your table as it has to mine.

Serves 2

Time:
40 minutes

Macros:
Under 550kcal,
26g protein per serving

2 skinless salmon fillets

½ teaspoon garlic granules

1 unwaxed lemon

320g (11¼oz) sheet of ready-rolled puff pastry

1 medium free-range egg, beaten

Salt and pepper

For the creamy leeks

2 teaspoons olive oil

1 large leek, trimmed, cleaned and finely sliced

1 garlic clove, minced

1 heaped teaspoon plain (all-purpose) flour

250ml (generous 1 cup) chicken stock

2 tablespoons half-fat crème fraîche

1 teaspoon Dijon mustard

2 handfuls of baby spinach leaves

30g (1oz) Parmesan cheese, grated

2 tablespoons chopped chives

- Preheat the oven to 200°C/180°C fan (400°F) Gas Mark 6. Line a baking tray with baking paper.

- Unroll the pastry and pat the salmon dry. Season the salmon with the garlic granules, some salt and pepper, a grating of lemon zest and a squeeze of lemon juice (keep the remaining for the creamy leeks).

- Lay the pastry out on the lined baking tray and place a salmon fillet on it. Cut around the salmon, leaving about a 2cm (¾ inch) border. Cut an identical sized piece from the pastry, then cut it into long strips. Brush the edges of the pastry base with beaten egg and start layering the strips over the salmon in a lattice pattern. Trim off any excess pastry and then repeat with the second salmon fillet and remaining pastry.

- Brush the pastry all over with beaten egg and bake in the oven for 20 minutes, or until the pastry is golden brown.

- While the salmon bakes, make the sauce. Heat the oil in a deep pan and sauté the leek for 5 minutes with a pinch of salt, being careful not to let it brown.

- Add the garlic and sauté for a few more minutes, then sprinkle in the flour and cook for 1 minute, stirring, before gradually whisking in the chicken stock. Allow it to simmer over a medium heat, stirring from time to time, for 5 minutes, until thickened. Stir in the crème fraîche, mustard and spinach, allowing the spinach to wilt.

- Finally, mix in the Parmesan, the chives, the remaining lemon zest from the reserved lemon, and a little squeeze of lemon juice. Adjust the seasoning as needed. The sauce should be thick enough to coat a spoon but remain somewhat runny.

- Serve the salmon en croûte on a bed of creamy leek sauce.

Chicken Katsu Curry

Serves 2

Time:
40 minutes

Macros:
Under 550kcal,
30g protein per serving

A balanced fakeaway favourite that you will love making at home. Easily adaptable to become vegetarian, you can simply use tofu slices and vegetable stock. Perfect for a Friday night in, full of warming spices with no compromise on flavour. Paired with a vibrant pickled cucumber salad, this really is just so good.

100g (½ cup) brown rice

2 boneless, skinless chicken breasts

1 medium free-range egg, beaten

1 teaspoon ginger and garlic paste

100g (2 cups) panko breadcrumbs

4 heaped tablespoons cornflour (cornstarch)

Spritz of neutral spray oil

Salt and pepper

For the cucumber pickle

½ cucumber, thinly sliced

100ml (scant ½ cup) rice vinegar

1 teaspoon toasted sesame oil

1 teaspoon caster (superfine) sugar

- Preheat the oven to 220°C/200°C fan (425°F) Gas Mark 7.

- Combine the cucumber pickle ingredients in a bowl and set aside to pickle.

- Cook the rice according to the packet instructions, then drain.

- Meanwhile, butterfly the chicken breasts by placing your hand on top of one. Use a sharp knife to slice horizontally into the thicker part, being careful not to cut all the way through. Open it up like a book, to resemble a butterfly. Repeat with the second breast and season both with salt and pepper.

- Prepare 3 shallow bowls: one with the beaten egg mixed with the garlic and ginger paste, one with the panko, and one with the cornflour, seasoned with salt and pepper. Lightly dust the chicken in the cornflour, dip into the egg mixture, and then firmly press into the panko, ensuring a thorough coating on all sides.

- Spray neutral oil on the coated chicken on both sides. Place on a baking tray and bake in the oven for 20–25 minutes, flipping halfway through, until golden and crisp.

- While the chicken is baking, make the sauce. Heat the oil in a saucepan over a medium heat and sauté the onion for about 5 minutes or until softened.

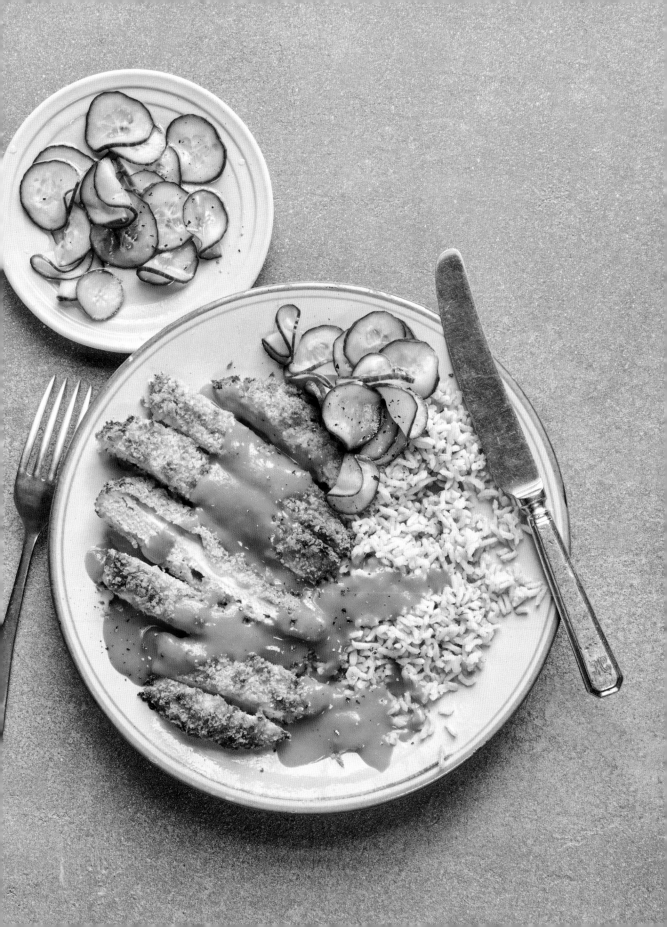

For the sauce

2 teaspoons olive oil

1 onion, finely chopped

2 teaspoons garlic and ginger paste

1 teaspoon medium curry powder

½ teaspoon ground turmeric

½ teaspoon ground star anise

15g (1¾ tablespoons) plain (all-purpose) flour

275ml (scant 1¼ cups) hot chicken stock, made with 1 stock cube

1 tablespoon tomato ketchup

1–2 teaspoons soft light brown sugar

- Add the ginger and garlic paste to the saucepan and fry for a few more seconds before adding the curry powder, turmeric and star anise. Season with salt and pepper and cook for another minute, then sprinkle in the flour and mix well.

- Gradually pour in the stock, stirring constantly. Add the tomato ketchup and brown sugar, then bring the mixture to a simmer. Cook for 5 minutes, stirring occasionally. Remove from the heat and cool slightly, then blend to a smooth consistency in a blender or food processor.

- Serve the panko-coated chicken with the pickled cucumber, a generous helping of the sauce and the cooked rice.

Chicken and Smoky Romesco

This dish is a consistent favourite among my friends, and it's not hard to see why. It's incredibly delicious yet simple to make, and is packed with health-promoting nutrients and heart-healthy monounsaturated fats from the extra virgin olive oil and hazelnuts. For the ultimate dinner, pair it with complex carbs from brown rice. Don't forget to save any leftover Romesco – it makes a great spread for toast or a tasty dip to enjoy throughout the week.

Serves 4

Time:
45 minutes

Macros:
Under 500kcal,
20g protein per serving

400g (14oz) skinless, boneless chicken thighs

1 tablespoon olive oil, plus extra for drizzling

1 teaspoon garlic granules

1 teaspoon onion powder

1 heaped teaspoon smoked paprika

1–2 large red (bell) pepper/s, cored, deseeded and cut into large chunks

2 banana shallots, halved lengthways

1 whole garlic bulb, halved horizontally

200g (generous 1 cup) brown rice

400ml (1⅔ cups) water

60g (½ cup) skin-on whole hazelnuts

Salt and pepper

To finish the Romesco

1–2 tablespoons sherry vinegar, to taste (or use red wine vinegar)

1 tablespoon tomato purée (paste)

1 teaspoon smoked paprika

1 tablespoon extra virgin olive oil

To serve

200g (7oz) French beans, topped and tailed

1 teaspoon olive oil

Handful of parsley leaves, chopped

Handful of basil leaves

Lemon wedges

- Preheat the oven to 220°C/200°C fan (425°F) Gas Mark 7.

- Toss the chicken thighs in the olive oil, garlic granules, onion powder, smoked paprika and some salt and pepper. Set aside.

- Place the red peppers and shallots face down in a baking dish. Add the garlic bulb halves, cut-side up, to the middle of the dish and drizzle with a little olive oil. Nestle the chicken thighs into the dish on top of the peppers and shallots.

- Roast in the oven for 20–25 minutes until the chicken is cooked through and golden and the peppers are soft.

- Meanwhile, in a pan, combine the rice and water. Stir with a fork to prevent clumping. Season with salt and pepper, then cover and bring to the boil. Reduce the heat to medium and cook for 12–15 minutes or until all the liquid has been absorbed and the rice is tender.

- Place the hazelnuts in a separate baking dish and roast in the oven for 5–7 minutes (this can be done at the same time as the chicken) until they release their nutty aroma.

- Remove the chicken thighs to a plate and cover in foil to keep them warm.

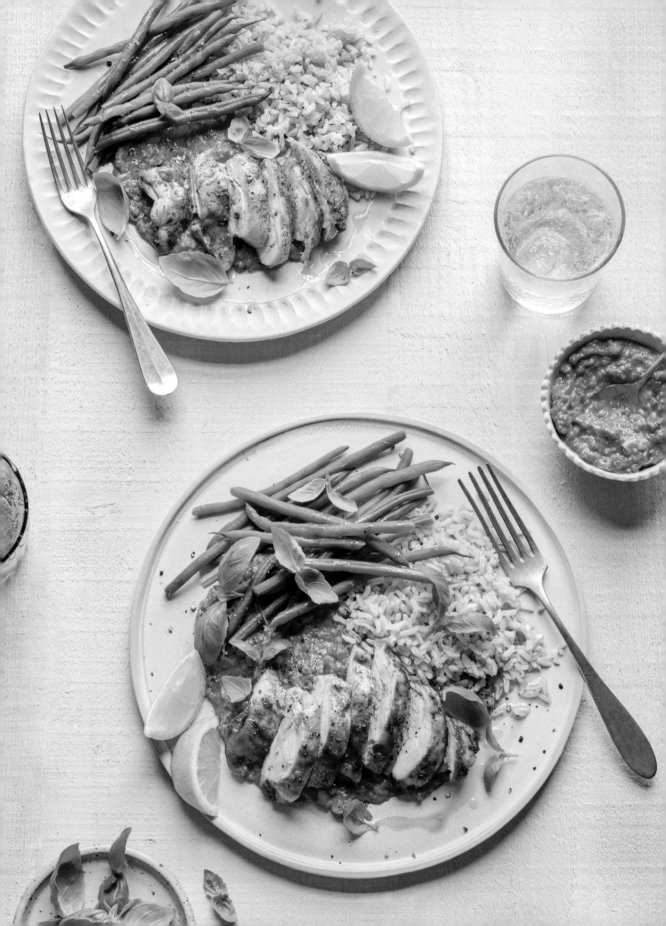

- To finish the Romesco, transfer the roasted peppers and shallots, 3–4 squeezed-out cloves of the roast garlic and the roasted hazelnuts to a blender (see note below on storing the leftover roast garlic). Add 1 tablespoon of the sherry vinegar, the tomato purée, smoked paprika, extra virgin olive oil and some salt and pepper to taste. Pulse a few times until you achieve a rough textural mix, retaining some of the texture of the hazelnuts. Taste and add more sherry vinegar, according to taste.

- Steam the French beans for 3 minutes, then toss them in the oil and parsley, with salt to taste.

- To serve, spread 2 tablespoons of Romesco onto each plate. Add a few spoonfuls of rice, some French beans and slices of chicken thigh. Garnish with basil leaves for a pop of colour, and serve with lemon wedges on the side.

Note:

Squeeze out the cloves of the garlic you aren't using, put into a small jar or airtight container and top with a little olive oil to cover. Refrigerate and use within 1 week – in pasta dishes, dressings or spreads.

Wholegrain Fish and Chips with Tartare Sauce

I love fish and chips. This is my take on the perfect midweek fish supper. Peas are a fantastic source of key energizing B vitamins, zinc and folate. Freezing peas actually helps lock in all of the goodness too. You can swap the cod for any fish you like in this recipe.

Serves 2

Time:
30 minutes

Macros:
Under 500kcal,
33g protein per serving

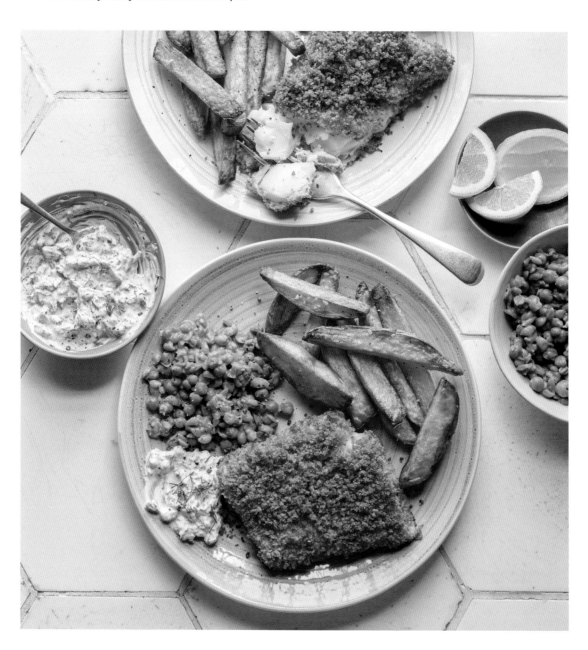

2 cod loins, about 130g (4½oz) each

80g (2¾oz) wholemeal (wholewheat) bread

2 teaspoons olive oil, plus extra for the potatoes

Zest of 1 unwaxed lemon

1 teaspoon garlic granules

250g (9oz) potatoes, cut into wedges

1 medium free-range egg

30g (4 tablespoons) plain (all-purpose) flour

Salt and pepper

Lemon wedges, to serve

For the tartare sauce

3–4 tablespoons thick natural yogurt (0% fat)

Juice of ½ lemon

4 gherkins, finely chopped, plus 2 teaspoons pickle juice from the jar

1 heaped tablespoon capers, chopped

½ teaspoon garlic paste

Handful of mixed dill and chives, finely chopped

For the peas

8–10 tablespoons frozen peas

½ vegetable stock cube, crumbled

1 tablespoon water

1 tablespoon half-fat crème fraîche

20g (¾oz) Parmesan cheese, grated

- Preheat the oven to 220°C/200°C fan (405°F) Gas Mark 7.

- Dry the cod well, season with salt and place in the refrigerator for 5 minutes while you prepare the breadcrumbs.

- In a food processor, blitz the bread into crumbs and then add to a frying pan over a medium heat with the olive oil, lemon zest, garlic granules and some salt and pepper. Fry, stirring, for around 3 minutes, until slightly golden brown, then tip into a shallow bowl.

- Toss your potato wedges in a little olive oil and some salt and pepper, spread out on a baking tray and bake in the oven for 25–30 minutes, until nice and roasted.

- Once the potatoes are in the oven, beat the egg in a second shallow bowl. Dust the cod with the flour to coat all sides, dip into the egg to coat then firmly press into the crumbs, covering all of the cod.

- Place on a separate baking tray and add to the oven alongside the potatoes when they have been in for 10 minutes. Bake for 15–20 minutes, depending on the thickness of your cod, until golden and crisp.

- Meanwhile, to make the tartare sauce, mix the yogurt with the lemon juice, the gherkins with their pickle juice, the capers, garlic paste, herbs and a pinch of salt. Taste and adjust, adding more salt, lemon juice or herbs if you wish.

- Tip the frozen peas straight into a frying pan with the crumbled stock cube and water and simmer over a medium-high heat for 2 minutes, then add in the crème fraîche and Parmesan. Season with a little salt and pepper and, using a fork, roughly mash. Taste and adjust the seasoning.

- Serve a portion of peas with the potatoes, crispy baked cod, a dollop of tartare sauce and a wedge of lemon on the side.

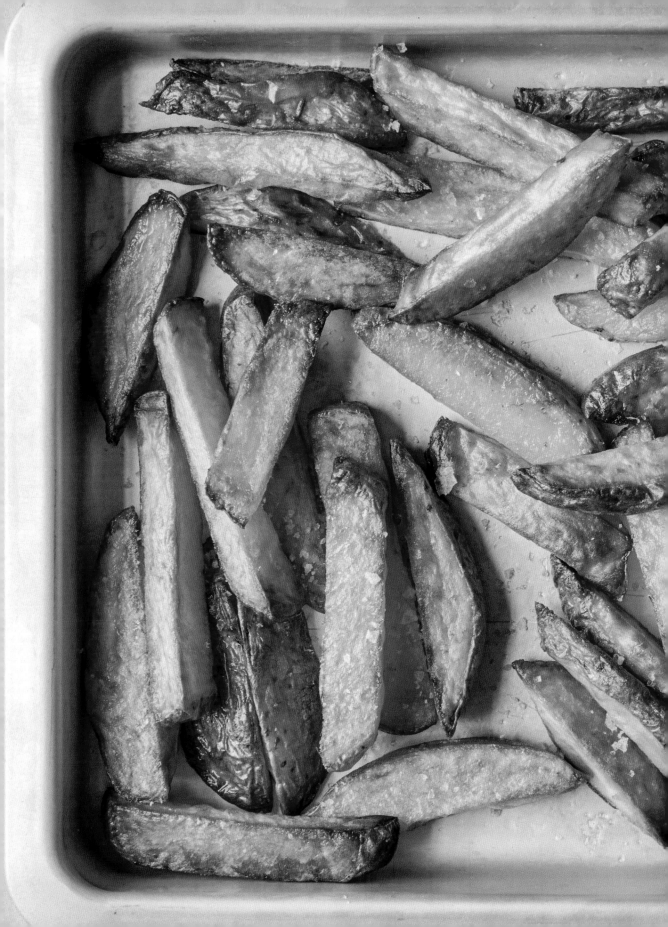

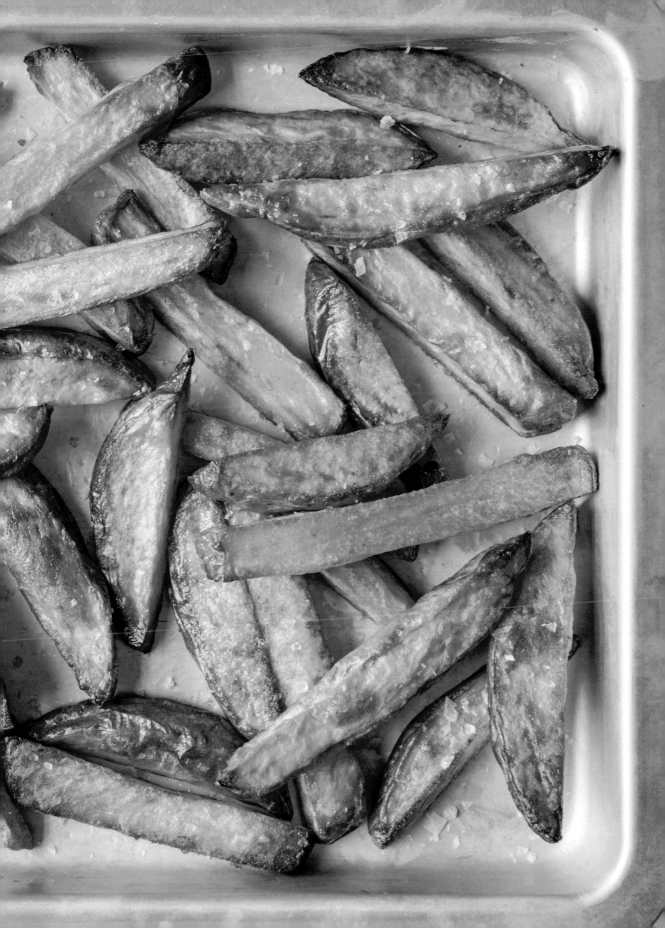

Roasted Tomato Soup with Giant Parmesan Croutons

Serves 2

Time:
55 minutes

Macros:
Under 300kcal,
6g protein per serving

Tomato soup has always been such a classic recipe that I couldn't resist including it in this book. It's pure comfort food, and the homemade giant cheesy croutons are perfect for mopping up every last bit.

300g (10½oz) ripe tomatoes, halved

½ red chilli, destemmed (omit if you don't like heat)

1 medium carrot, roughly chopped

1 red onion, roughly chopped

1 medium whole garlic bulb, halved horizontally

2 teaspoons extra virgin olive oil

Small bunch of thyme, leaves stripped

400g (14oz) can of good-quality tomatoes (I use whole cherry tomatoes for sweetness)

1 chicken or vegetable stock cube

1 teaspoon honey

1 heaped tablespoon half-fat crème fraîche

Salt and pepper

Handful of basil leaves, to finish

For the croutons

150g (5½oz) sourdough, cut into large squares or pieces

½ teaspoon garlic granules

2 teaspoons olive oil

Parmesan cheese, for grating

- Preheat the oven to 220°C/200°C fan (425°F) Gas Mark 7.

- In a deep baking tray (deep enough to hold the liquid), place the halved tomatoes, chilli, carrot, red onion and garlic bulb halves. Drizzle with the extra virgin olive oil, sprinkle with the thyme and season with salt and pepper, then roast in the oven for 25 minutes, until golden.

- Add the canned tomatoes to the tray, then fill the empty can with water, pour it into the tray and crumble in the stock cube. Turn the oven down to 190°C/170°C fan (375°F) Gas Mark 5 and roast for another 15 minutes.

- Meanwhile, toss the sourdough pieces in the garlic granules, some salt and the olive oil and spread out on a lined baking tray. Grate a generous amount of Parmesan over them and bake in the oven for 5–10 minutes until golden. Remove and set aside.

- Remove the garlic bulb halves from the deep baking tray and squeeze the contents of 3–4 garlic cloves back into the tray (see note on page 141 on storing leftover roast garlic). Add the honey and crème fraîche and then blend to a smooth soup in a food processor or blender. Season with salt and pepper if needed. If the soup is too thick, you can loosen it with some more stock. Check the temperature and reheat on the hob if needed. Finish by stirring in the basil leaves.

- Serve the soup in bowls, top with the golden croutons and enjoy!

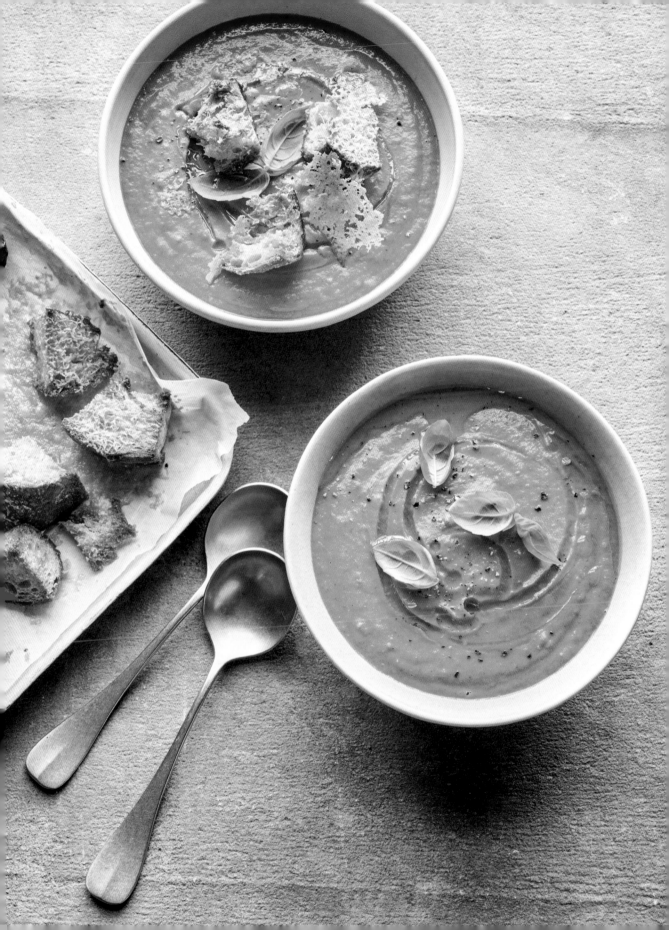

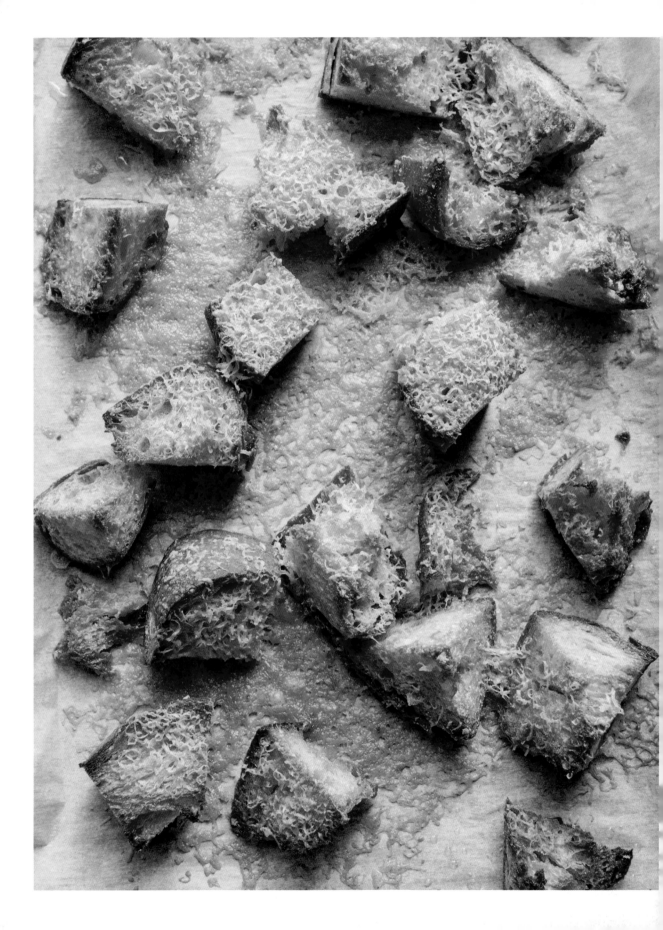

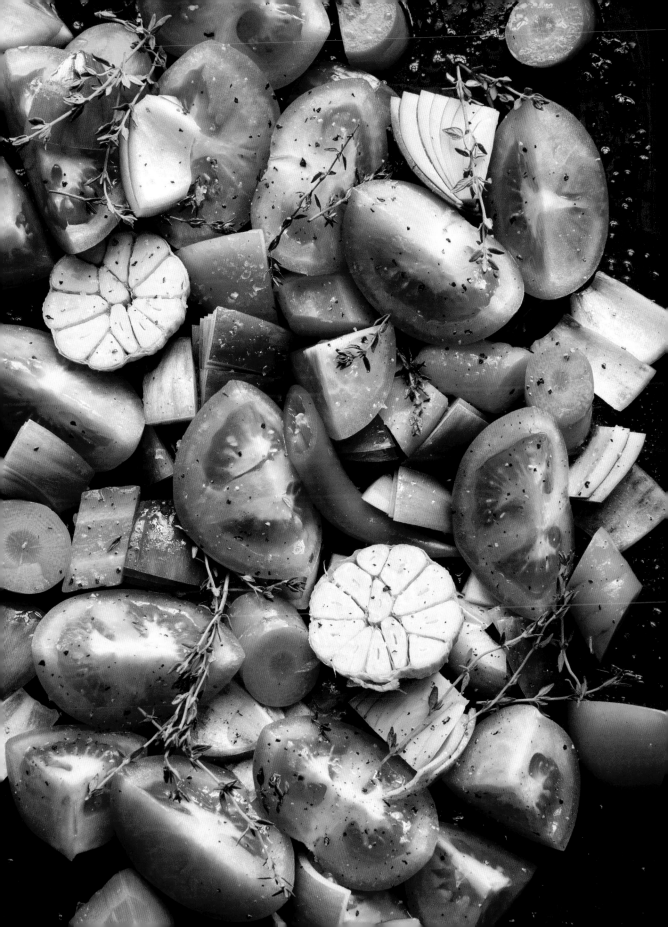

Creamy Parmesan Chickpeas with Pickled Chilli

Serves 2

Time:
35 minutes

Macros:
Under 300kcal,
15g protein per serving

Humble chickpeas cook down with onions, garlic, Parmesan and spinach to form an unctuous and creamy base to top with either grilled chicken breast, fish or a vegetarian/vegan substitute (if cooking as a vegetarian or vegan dish, the Parmesan will also need to be substituted). It's satisfying, simple and transforms a simple can of chickpeas into a total crowd-pleaser. I often keep my leftover Parmesan rinds just for this recipe!

2 teaspoons olive oil

1 shallot, finely diced

1 carrot, very finely diced

1 celery stick, very finely diced

1 garlic clove, minced

400g (14oz) can of good-quality chickpeas (or the ones in glass jars are incredible and worth trying to find)

1 chicken or veg stock cube, crumbled

50g (1¾oz) Parmesan cheese, grated, plus the end wedge (including the rind), and extra grated Parmesan to serve

Zest of ½ unwaxed lemon

2 handfuls of baby spinach leaves

Salt and pepper

For the pickled chilli

1 red chilli, deseeded and thinly sliced

150ml (⅔ cup) white wine vinegar

1 tablespoon caster (superfine) sugar

- For the pickled chilli, add the chilli slices to a bowl and pour over the vinegar to cover. Stir in the sugar and leave to one side.

- Heat the olive oil in a saucepan and add the shallot, carrot, celery and garlic with a pinch of salt. Sauté over a medium heat for 5 minutes or until the vegetables soften.

- Tip in the entire contents of the chickpea can, including the brine. Refill the can with 200ml (scant 1 cup) of water and add to the pan.

- Stir in the stock cube, Parmesan rind wedge and a generous crack of black pepper.

- Let the mixture simmer for 15 minutes, stirring now and then. It should reduce to thicken but remain saucy. If it thickens too much, add a bit more water.

- Take off the heat, discard the Parmesan rind and grate in the lemon zest.

- Gradually whisk in the grated Parmesan, stirring constantly for a smooth, thick sauce. Adjust the seasoning with more Parmesan, and salt and pepper to taste, then stir in the spinach until wilted.

- Finely dice 1 tablespoon of the pickled chilli slices and fold into the mix. Serve with a sprinkle of extra pickled chilli and a little flurry of Parmesan.

- Pair with a protein of your choice when serving.

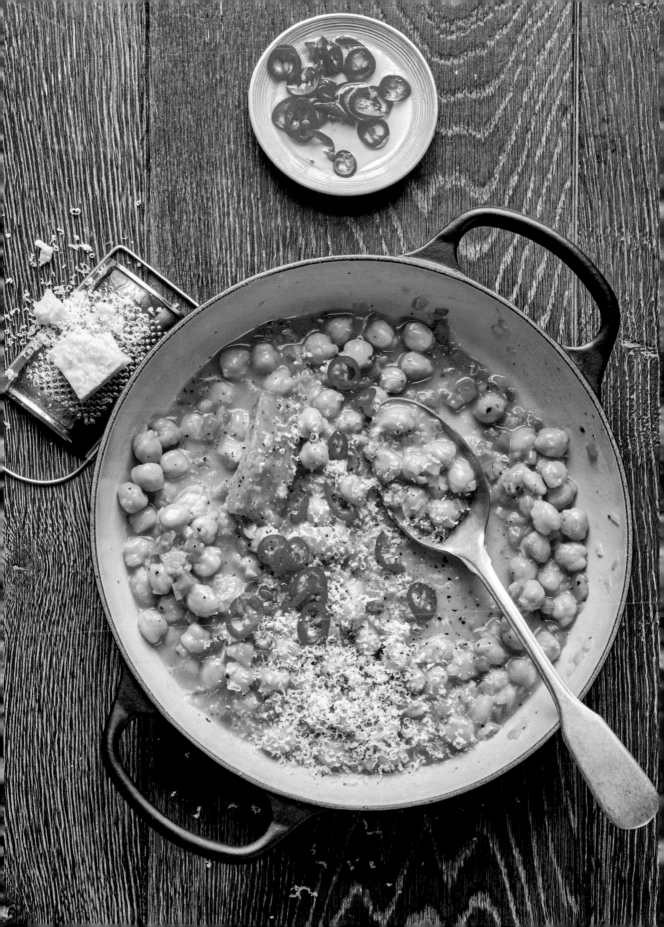

Italian Sausage and Broccoli Pasta

This is one of my favourite pasta dishes – a nod to all the flavours of the traditional Italian sausage pasta but with a few twists to lighten it up and make it a balanced midweek meal. I make this nearly every week when I want something quick but satisfying. You can adapt it for vegetarians by swapping the Parmesan and chicken sausages for vegetarian alternatives and using a tablespoon of chopped capers instead of the anchovies.

Serves 2

Time:
25 minutes

Macros:
Under 632kcal, 40g protein per serving

150g (5½oz) dried pasta of choice
(I like wholewheat fusilli or spaghetti)

5 chicken sausages, skins removed (I use Heck)

2 tablespoons olive oil

½ red onion, finely diced

1 heaped teaspoon fennel seeds, coarsely ground

2 anchovies in oil, drained and chopped

2 garlic cloves, finely diced

½ red chilli, deseeded and finely diced

2 tablespoons water

200g (7oz) Tenderstem broccoli,
cut into 2.5cm (1 inch) pieces

150g (⅔ cup) half-fat crème fraîche

Zest of 1 unwaxed lemon, plus lemon wedges to serve

60g (2¼oz) Parmesan cheese, grated

1 tablespoon chopped parsley, plus extra to serve

Salt and pepper

- Cook the pasta in a pan of boiling salted water until al dente, then drain and set aside.

- Meanwhile, using your hands, break up the sausages into small, rough pieces.

- Heat the olive oil in a frying pan and brown the sausage pieces over a medium heat for 3–4 minutes until they have some colour. Remove to a plate using a slotted spoon, then add the red onion, fennel seeds, anchovies, garlic, chilli and 1 teaspoon of pepper to the pan. Sauté for 5 minutes, adding 1 tablespoon of the water to help lift all the flavours from the bottom of the pan.

- Add the broccoli pieces to the pan, mix well and cook until softened but still with bite, adding the remaining 1 tablespoon of water to create steam to speed this up.

- Stir in the browned sausage pieces, drained pasta, the crème fraîche, lemon zest, Parmesan and parsley. Season to taste and serve with extra parsley, and lemon wedges on the side.

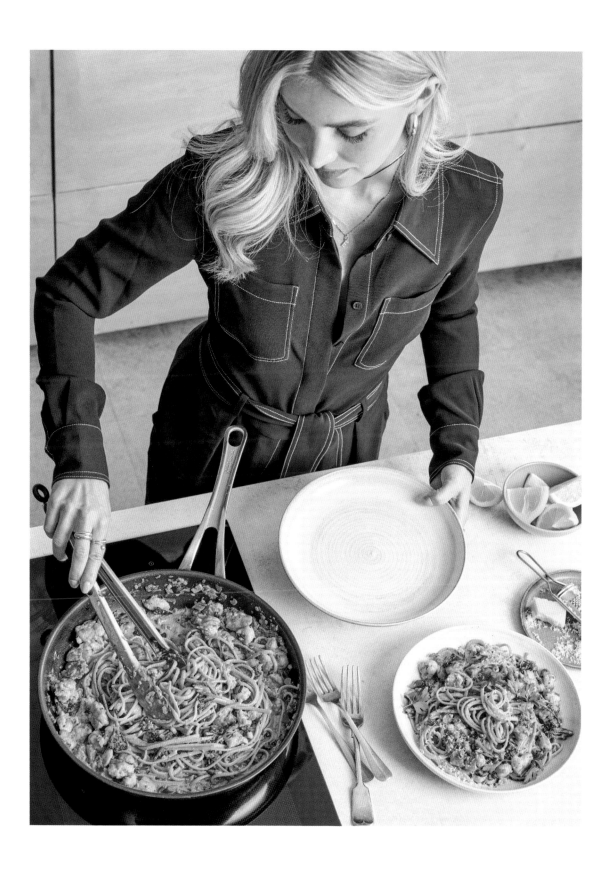

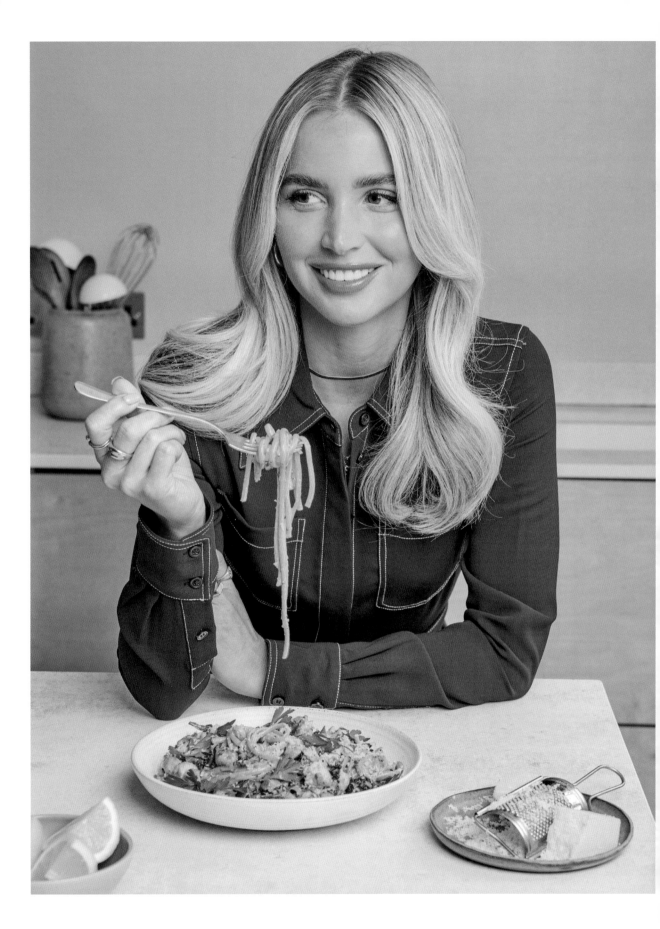

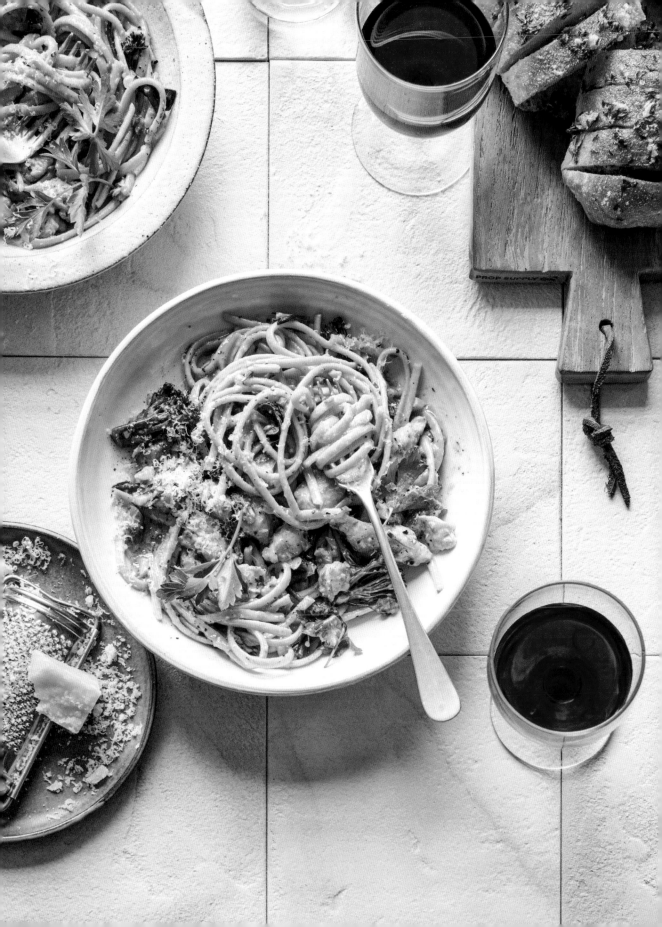

Thai Chicken and Butternut Soup

Serves 4

Time:
30 minutes

Macros:
Under 420kcal, 21g
protein per serving

An aromatic red Thai soup that feels hearty but balanced. Packed full of vegetables and vibrancy with all the bright flavours we all know and love from Thai cuisine. Use full-fat coconut milk for richness, and finish with a scattering of fresh coriander.

2 teaspoons olive oil

2 garlic cloves, chopped

½ red chilli, deseeded and diced

1 red (bell) pepper, cored, deseeded and chopped

1 teaspoon ginger paste

Small bunch of coriander (cilantro), stems chopped, leaves reserved separately

2 tablespoons red Thai curry paste

400g (14oz) can of coconut milk

1 chicken stock cube, crumbled

1 tablespoon fish sauce

1 teaspoon honey

500g (1lb 2oz) diced butternut squash

300g (10½oz) cooked chicken meat, shredded

Juice of ½ lime

Salt and pepper

- Heat the olive oil in a large saucepan over a medium heat. Add the garlic, chilli, red pepper, ginger paste, chopped coriander stems and curry paste and cook for 2–3 minutes until the aromas are released.

- Pour in the coconut milk, then refill the can twice with water and add this too. Add the stock cube, fish sauce, honey and the diced butternut. Turn down the heat to low-medium and simmer for 15 minutes, until the butternut is soft.

- Using a stick blender, blend to a smooth soup.

- Add the shredded chicken and heat gently for 2–3 minutes, then finish with the lime juice, taste and season if needed, scatter over the coriander leaves and serve.

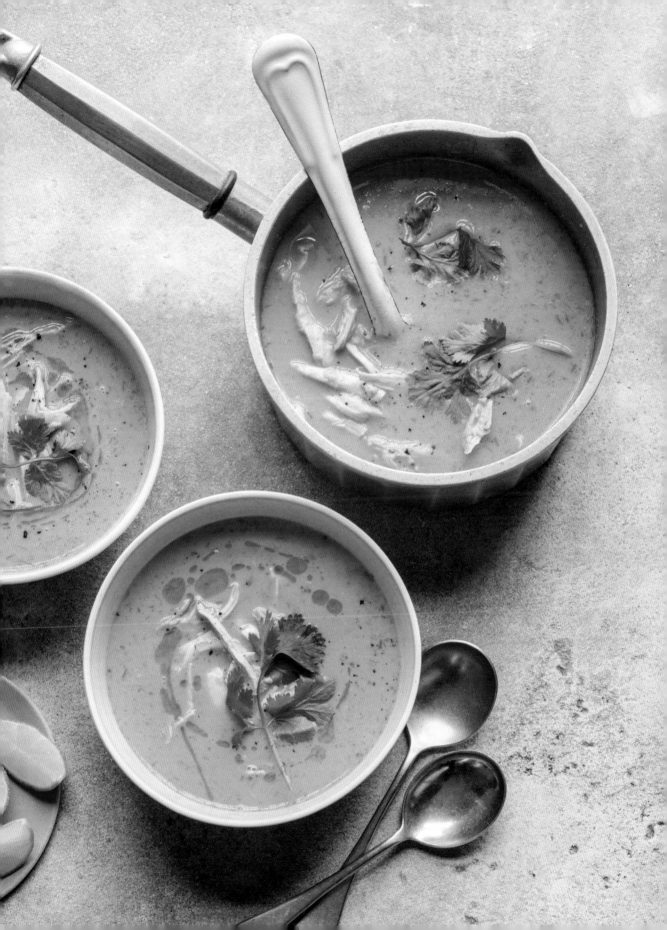

Spiced Turkey Koftas with Tabbouleh and Mint Yogurt

Serves 4

Time:
30 minutes

Macros:
Under 400kcal,
47g protein per serving

My spiced turkey koftas are loaded with courgette, lemon zest and one of my favourite spice blends, za'atar. I pair them with a refreshing tabbouleh salad made of quinoa, cucumber, tomatoes, red onion, pomegranate seeds and parsley, finished with a dollop of tangy mint yogurt for a wholesome and flavour-packed meal.

Olive oil, for cooking and brushing

Salt and pepper

For the koftas

1 courgette (zucchini), grated

500g (1lb 2oz) lean minced (ground) turkey

2 tablespoons each of chopped mint and parsley

4 tablespoons fresh wholemeal (wholewheat) breadcrumbs

1 medium free-range egg

Zest of 1 unwaxed lemon

1 heaped tablespoon za'atar spice mix

1 teaspoon garlic granules

For the mint yogurt

200g (scant 1 cup) thick natural yogurt (0% fat)

1 tablespoon chopped mint

Juice of ½ lemon

½ teaspoon garlic granules

For the tabbouleh

250g (9oz) cooked quinoa

½ cucumber, deseeded and diced

2 large tomatoes, deseeded and diced

½ red onion, finely diced

80g (2¾oz) pomegranate seeds

2 large handfuls of parsley, roughly chopped

Juice of ½ lemon

2 teaspoons extra virgin olive oil

- Preheat the oven to 200°C/180°C fan (400°F) Gas Mark 6.

- Heat 1 teaspoon of olive oil in a frying pan over a medium heat, add the grated courgette and a pinch of salt and sweat for 2 minutes or until softened. Set aside to cool slightly.

- In a bowl, combine the mint yogurt ingredients and set aside.

- In a large separate bowl, combine the cooked courgette with the remaining kofta ingredients and a generous pinch of salt and pepper, mixing well. Using your hands, shape the mixture into 12 sausage-like koftas and lightly brush with oil.

- Heat a dry frying pan over a medium-high heat, add the koftas and fry, turning, for 5 minutes, to brown on all sides. Transfer to a baking dish and finish cooking in the oven for 5 minutes, until cooked through.

- Meanwhile, for the tabbouleh, combine the quinoa, cucumber, tomatoes, red onion and pomegranate seeds in a dish. Add the parsley, lemon juice and extra virgin olive oil, and season to taste.

- Serve 3 koftas per plate, accompanied by some tabbouleh and a dollop of the mint yogurt.

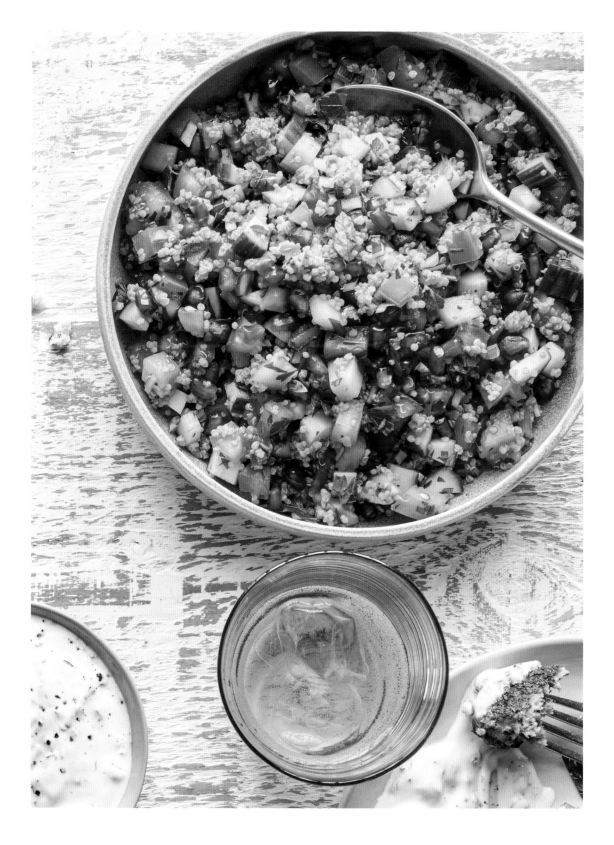

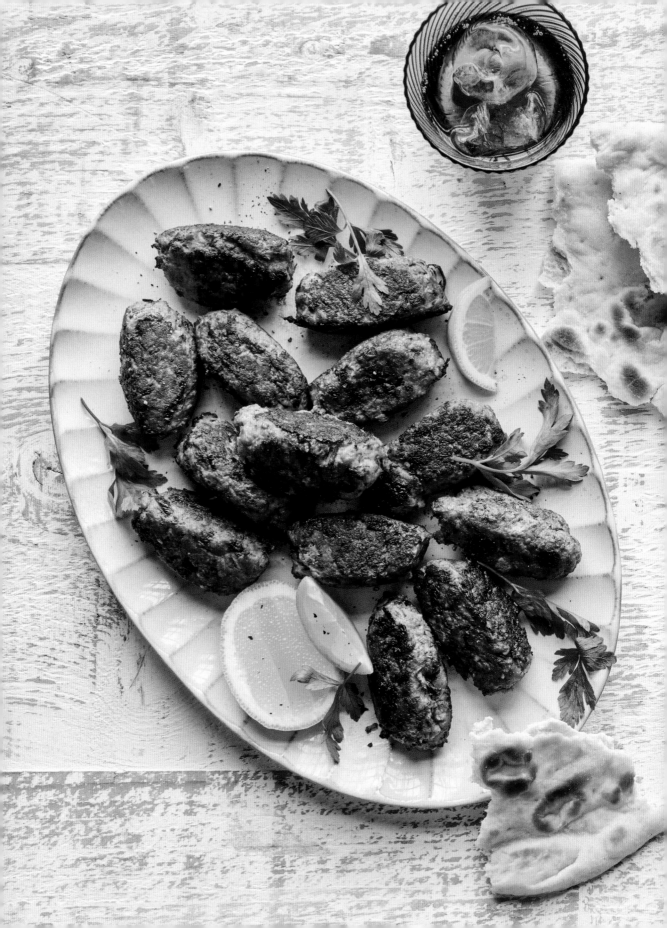

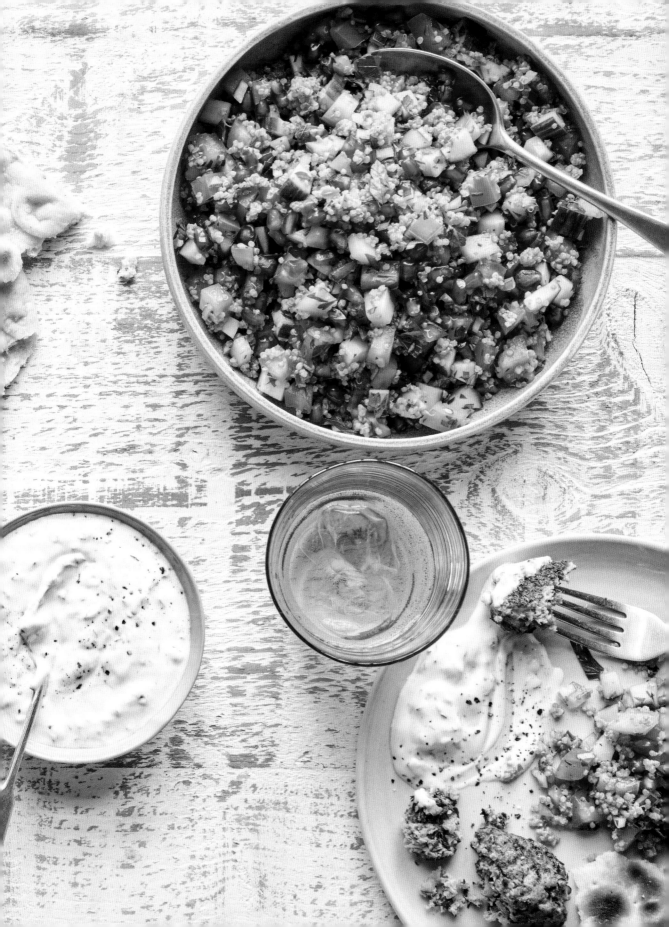

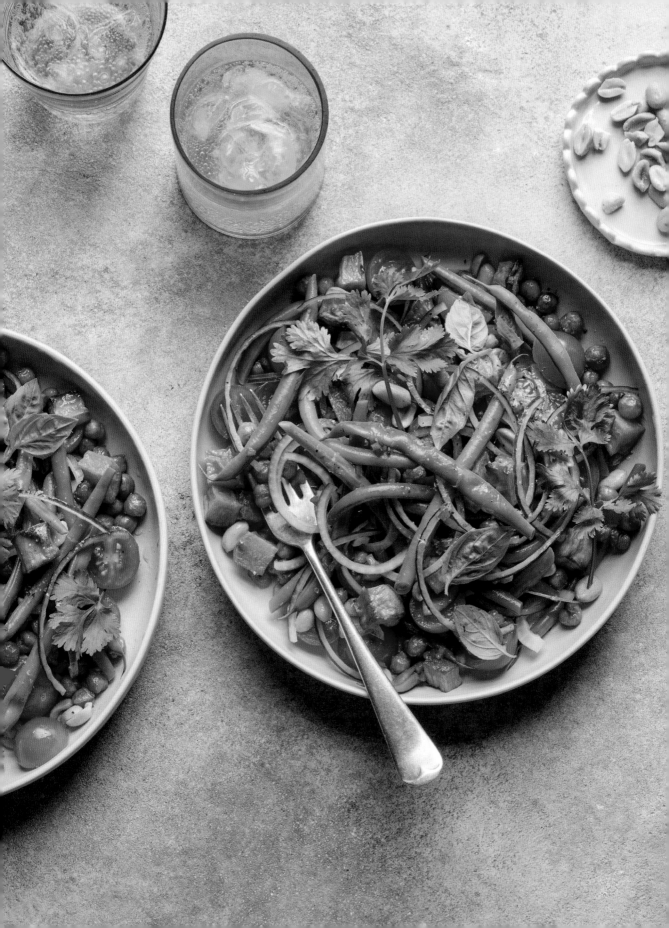

Hot and Sour
Thai Bowl

This salad offers the perfect balance of sweet, sour, hot and salty. Guaranteed to satisfy with its blend of slow-release carbs, filling protein and spice. The addition of sweet potato not only boosts fibre but also provides a source of vitamin A, which is one of my favourite skin-supporting ingredients.

Serves 2

Time:
30 minutes

Macros:
Under 400kcal,
10g protein per serving

300g (10½oz) sweet potato, peeled and cut into small cubes

400g (14oz) can of chickpeas, drained, rinsed and dried

2 teaspoons olive oil

1 teaspoon cornflour (cornstarch)

1 teaspoon garlic granules

200g (7oz) French beans, topped and tailed

1 red onion, thinly sliced

Small handful of coriander (cilantro) leaves, torn

2 large handfuls of cherry tomatoes, halved

3 tablespoons roasted salted peanuts

Salt and pepper

For the dressing

1 heaped teaspoon honey

Zest and juice of 1 lime

1 tablespoon rice vinegar

¼ red chilli, deseeded and finely diced

¼ teaspoon garlic granules

2 teaspoons toasted sesame oil

2 tablespoons fish sauce

Small handful of mint leaves

- Preheat the oven to 210°C/190°C fan (410°F) Gas Mark 6½.

- Mix together all the dressing ingredients in a bowl and set aside to let the flavours meld.

- Spread the sweet potato and chickpeas out on a baking tray. Add the olive oil, cornflour and garlic granules, with salt and pepper to taste, and mix to coat, then spread out again. Bake in the oven for 20–25 minutes until golden, stirring from time to time.

- Meanwhile, bring a pan of salted water to the boil. Blanch the French beans for 3 minutes, then drain and immediately run them under cold water to halt the cooking process.

- Remove the baked sweet potato and chickpeas from the oven and set them aside to cool slightly.

- In a large mixing bowl, combine the red onion, coriander, blanched French beans, roasted sweet potato and chickpeas, cherry tomatoes and salted peanuts.

- Pour the dressing over the salad, toss well to combine and serve.

Harissa Roasted Red Pepper Immunity Soup

I adore this Harissa Roasted Red Pepper Immunity Soup. It's quick and easy to make and is packed full of immune-supporting goodness. If you're feeling run-down or under the weather, this soup is for you. Some people might not have cooked with harissa paste, but a jar can last a long time in your refrigerator. It offers a wonderful warming flavour and is available in most supermarkets.

Serves 2

Time:
30 minutes

Macros:
Under 350kcal,
9g protein per serving

---

2 teaspoons olive oil

1 red onion, diced

Small bunch of basil, leaves and stems chopped separately, plus extra leaves to serve

1 teaspoon chopped garlic

1 tablespoon harissa paste, plus extra for spreading

1 tablespoon sun-dried tomato paste

450g (1lb) jar of roasted red (bell) peppers, drained

1 chicken stock cube, crumbled

40g (1½oz) feta cheese, crumbled, plus extra to serve

20g (¾oz) Parmesan cheese, grated

2 slices of sourdough or bread of choice

Salt and pepper

Dried chilli flakes, to serve

- Heat the olive oil in a deep saucepan over a medium heat, add the red onion, chopped basil stems and a pinch of salt and sauté for about 5 minutes until softened.

- Add the garlic, harissa paste, sun-dried tomato paste and drained red peppers. Mix well and cook for 2 minutes.

- Pour in enough boiling water to cover the red peppers by about 1cm (½ inch). Add the stock cube and allow the mixture to simmer gently for 10 minutes.

- Stir in the feta and chopped basil leaves, then season with pepper. Blend in a food processor or blender until smooth.

- To make the toast, sprinkle the Parmesan into a cold nonstick frying pan. Spread a little harissa paste over the sourdough slices and then press them down into the grated Parmesan in the pan. Place the pan over a medium heat, then pan-fry for 4–5 minutes, until golden and crisp. Flip and cook the other side for a few more minutes.

- Serve the soup with an extra sprinkle of feta and basil leaves, and a touch of chilli flakes for added heat, with the golden Parmesan toast on the side.

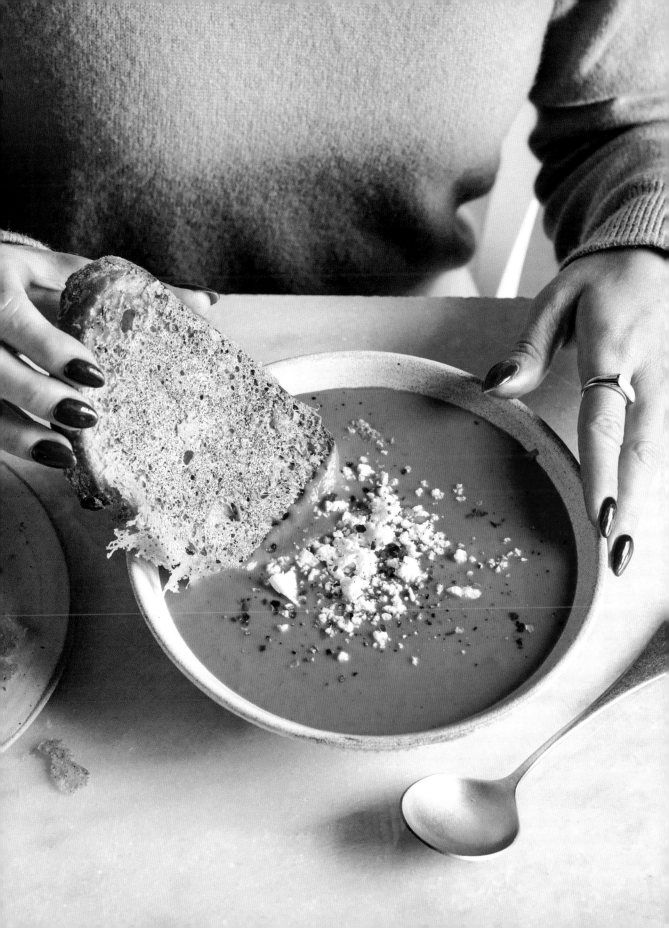

168–191

Sweet

168   Oaty Date Banoffee Pie

170   Single Serve Peach Cobbler

173   Flourless Orange Almond Cake

176   Dark Chocolate and Olive Oil Antioxidant Torte

181   Greek Yogurt Roasted Strawberry Eton Mess

184   High Fibre Apple and Berry Crumble

186   Bitter Lemon Tart

188   Victoria Sponge

191   Gut Food Lemon Drizzle Loaf

Oaty Date Banoffee Pie

Serves 12

Time:
35 minutes, plus
cooling time

Macros:
Under 300kcal,
5g protein per serving

A play on a banoffee pie but with a nutrient-dense oat and sunflower seed base, a fibre-rich Medjool date tahini caramel, finished off with sliced banana and a light whipped cream topping. It's a full showstopper and is always a crowd-pleaser whenever I make it for friends. You can store this in an airtight container in the refrigerator for up to 3 days.

For the date caramel

200g (7oz) pitted Medjool dates

1 heaped teaspoon tahini

1 teaspoon vanilla extract

Pinch of sea salt

3½–5 tablespoons almond milk

For the oat crust base

100g (¾ cup) sunflower seeds

250g (scant 2 cups) rolled oats

Pinch of sea salt

80ml (⅔ cup) maple syrup

60g (4 tablespoons) unsalted butter

For the topping

2 large bananas, cut into 2cm (¾ inch)-thick slices

100g (½ cup) whipping (heavy whipping) cream

Unsweetened cocoa powder, for dusting

- Preheat the oven to 190°C/170°C fan (375°F) Gas Mark 5. Line a 23cm (9 inch) loose-bottomed tart tin (pan) with nonstick baking paper.

- Begin by soaking the dates. Place them in a small bowl, cover with hot water from a recently boiled kettle and let them soak for 10 minutes, then drain and set to one side.

- Meanwhile, for the base, put the sunflower seeds, oats and salt in a food processor and blend until the mixture reaches a sandy texture and the sunflower seeds have broken down. Add the maple syrup and butter to the oat mixture and pulse until combined and the mixture begins to clump together. If necessary, add a little water, a tablespoon at a time, until it binds together.

- Press the mixture into the lined tart tin, gently prick the base with a fork and bake in the oven for 15 minutes. Remove and allow to cool.

- For the date caramel, in a blender or food processor, blend the drained soaked dates with the tahini, vanilla and salt, adding enough almond milk to achieve a smooth, thick consistency.

- Once the tart base has cooled, spread the date caramel over it. Lightly press the banana slices into the caramel until covered.

- Place in the refrigerator to set for 5 minutes.

- Meanwhile, in a mixing bowl, whip the cream until stiff but spreadable. Spoon and spread the cream over the banana slices and finish by sifting a light dusting of cocoa powder over the top before serving.

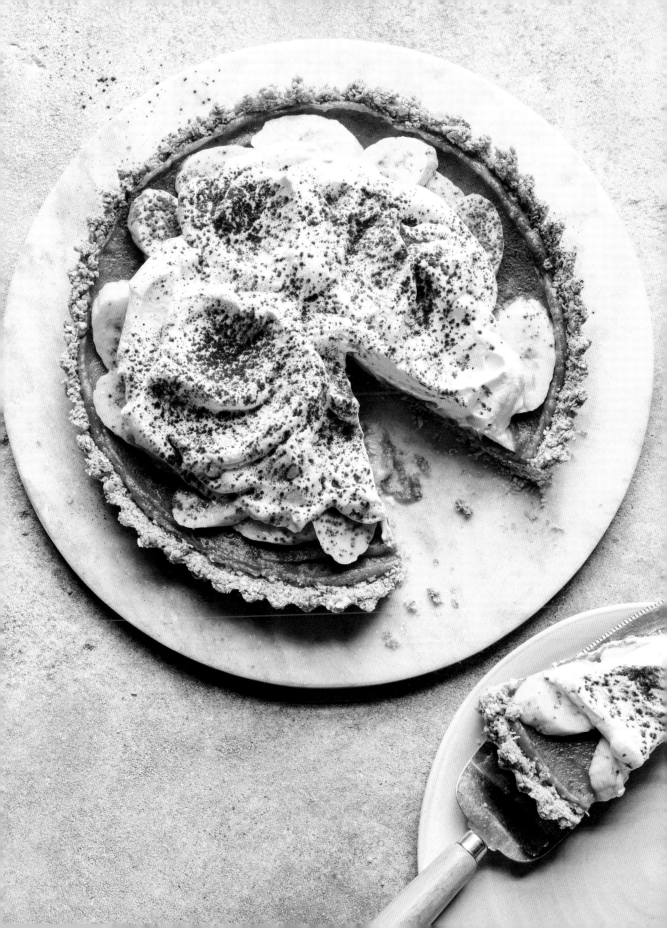

Single Serve
Peach Cobbler

This single serve plant-based dessert is the perfect thing to turn to when you want something healthy and quick to satisfy your sweet tooth. A super-quick 6-ingredient cobbler topping made with peanut butter creates these gorgeous crunchy and crumbly clusters.

Serves 1

Time:
30 minutes

Macros:
Under 250kcal,
5g protein

30g (2 heaped tablespoons) rolled oats

1 teaspoon smooth peanut butter

1 heaped teaspoon honey

1 teaspoon vanilla extract

Small pinch of salt

1 ripe peach, halved, pitted and diced

- Preheat the oven to 190°C/170°C fan (375°F) Gas Mark 5.

- In a bowl, mix the oats, peanut butter, honey, vanilla and salt and rub together with your fingertips until combined.

- Place the diced peach in a ramekin and top with the oat mix, pressing down slightly.

- Bake in the oven for 20–25 minutes, until the top is golden and the peach is softened.

- Serve with natural yogurt or ice cream.

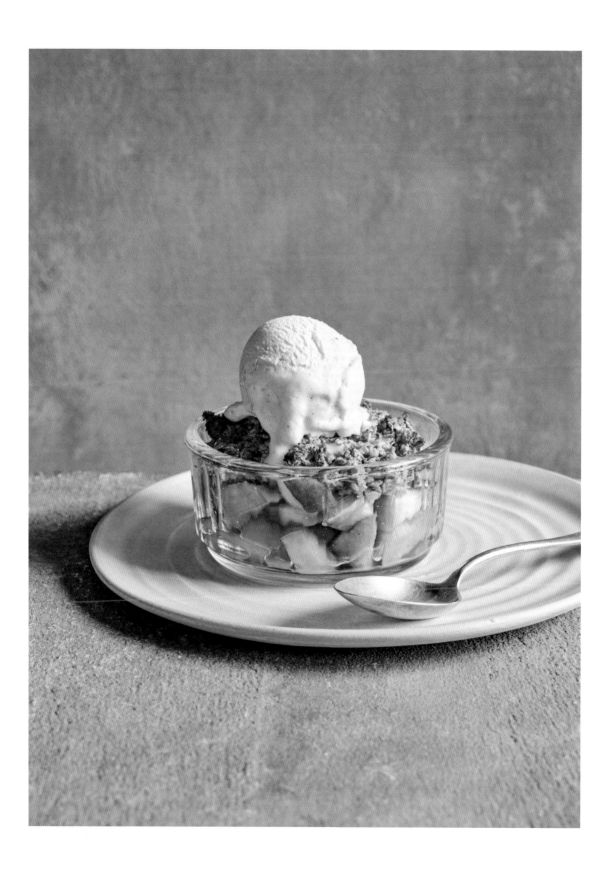

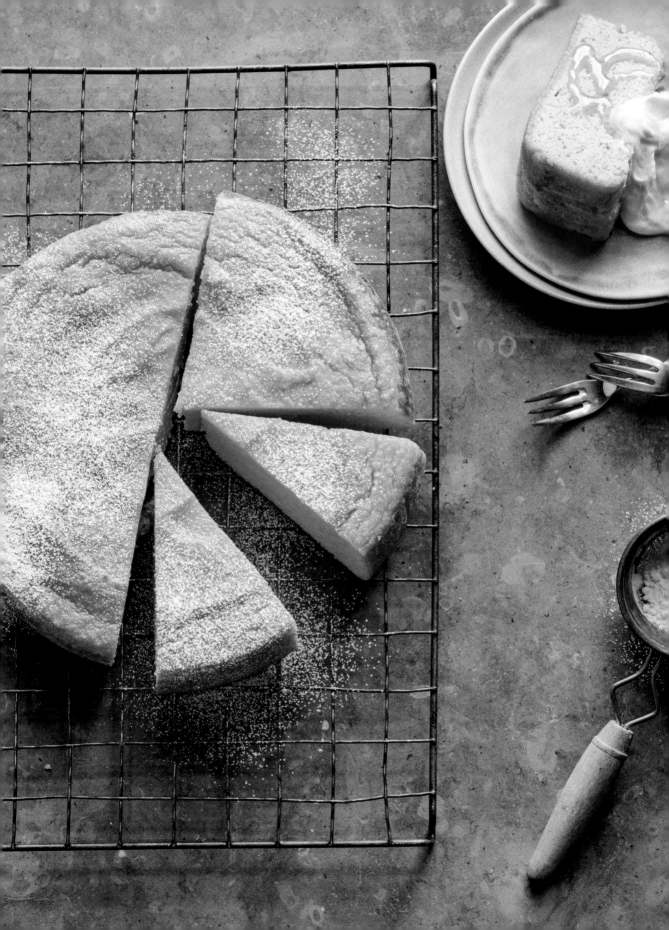

Flourless Orange Almond Cake

Serves 10

Time:
1 hour 15 minutes
(plus 1 hour to cook
the oranges)

Macros:
Under 250kcal,
3g protein per serving

A refreshing, ultra-moist, nutrient-rich cake that marries the citrusy brightness of oranges with the rich depth of almonds. This flourless treat is not only delicious but also offers a nutritious and gluten-free alternative for those looking for a sticky and rich cake. Almonds also provide a dose of healthy fats and antioxidants. Enjoy with a big dollop of thick natural yogurt and a drizzle of honey, or keep in an airtight container in the refrigerator for up to 5 days.

2 large oranges

6 medium free-range eggs

150g (¾ cup) caster (superfine) sugar

1 teaspoon vanilla extract

225g (2¼ cups) ground almonds

1 teaspoon gluten-free baking powder

Icing (confectioners') sugar, for dusting (optional)

Thick natural yogurt and honey, to serve

- Cook the whole, unpeeled oranges in a pan of boiling water, ensuring they are fully submerged, for about 1 hour. Drain and let them cool.

- Once cooled, peel the oranges, separating the peel and the flesh. Discard any seeds and excess pith. Blend the flesh and peel in a blender until you get a smooth purée.

- Preheat the oven to 190°C/170°C fan (375°F) Gas Mark 5. Line a 20cm (8 inch) cake tin (pan) with nonstick baking paper.

- In a large bowl, whisk the eggs and sugar together until well combined and slightly fluffy. Tip in the orange purée, vanilla extract, ground almonds and baking powder, and use a large metal spoon to fold together and combine.

- Tip the mixture into the lined tin and bake in the oven for about 1 hour, until a cocktail stick (toothpick) inserted into the middle comes out clean, keeping a watch that the top doesn't brown too quickly. If it does, place a piece of foil loosely over the top.

- Remove from the oven and let the cake set in the tin for 20 minutes. Turn it out, remove the lining and flip the cake on to a wire rack to cool. Feel free to brush with a little honey and dust over some icing sugar. Serve each slice with a dollop of yogurt drizzled with honey.

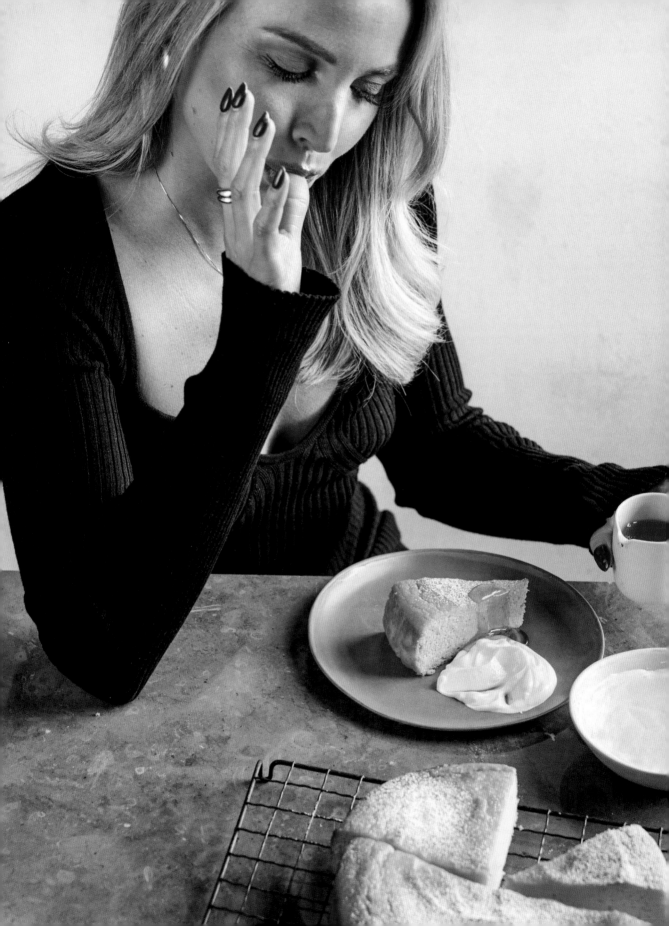

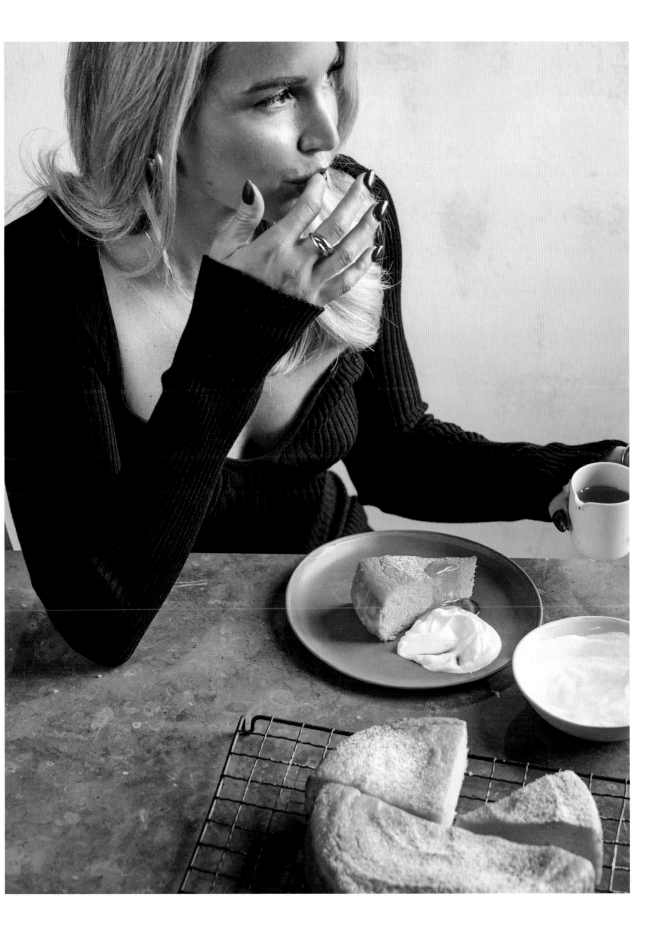

Dark Chocolate and Olive Oil Antioxidant Torte

Serves 12

Time:
1 hour 10 minutes, plus cooling time

Macros:
Under 350kcal, 2g protein per serving

A rich antioxidant-packed torte that is perfectly fudgy and makes the ultimate decadent slice. Full of heart-healthy olive oil and rich cocoa, it's not too sweet but it's a dessert that makes a wonderful treat, with a few of those extra nutritional benefits. Blending the hazelnuts with the skin on into a flour boosts the fibre content and helps slow down any sugar spikes too. You can keep your torte in an airtight container in the refrigerator for up to 3 days.

150g (scant 1¼ cups) skin-on whole hazelnuts

50g (½ cup) unsweetened cocoa powder

125ml (½ cup) boiling water

2 teaspoons vanilla extract

150g (¾ cup) caster (superfine) sugar

130ml (generous ½ cup) extra virgin olive oil, plus extra for greasing

3 medium free-range eggs, at room temperature

½ teaspoon bicarbonate of soda (baking soda)

Pinch of salt

For the chocolate ganache topping

100g (3½oz) dark chocolate (70% cocoa content) roughly chopped

5 tablespoons hazelnut milk

A little orange zest (optional)

- Preheat the oven to 190°C/170°C fan (375°F) Gas Mark 5. Lightly oil a 21cm (8¼ inch) springform cake tin (pan) and line the base with nonstick baking paper.

- Place the hazelnuts on a baking tray and roast in the oven for 10 minutes until they give off a gorgeous nutty aroma and are looking toasted. Allow to cool, then in a food processor or blender, blend into a flour and set aside. Keep the oven on.

- While the hazelnuts are cooling, sift the cocoa powder into a bowl and mix with the boiling water to form a paste. Stir in the vanilla extract and let cool.

- In a large bowl, whisk the sugar, olive oil and eggs together for about 5 minutes until fluffy and pale. Gradually stir in the cocoa mixture, then fold in the bicarb, salt and hazelnut flour.

- Tip the batter into the prepared tin and bake in the oven for 35–40 minutes, keeping it slightly undercooked for a fudgier texture. The torte should be set at the sides with a slightly moist centre.

- Allow the torte to cool in its tin for 10 minutes, then transfer to a wire rack to cool completely.

- To make the ganache topping, place the chopped chocolate in a heatproof bowl. Heat the hazelnut milk in a pan until warm but not simmering, then pour over the chocolate. Let it sit for a minute, then stir until smooth. Feel free to grate in some orange zest if you wish. Spread the ganache over the cooled torte and serve.

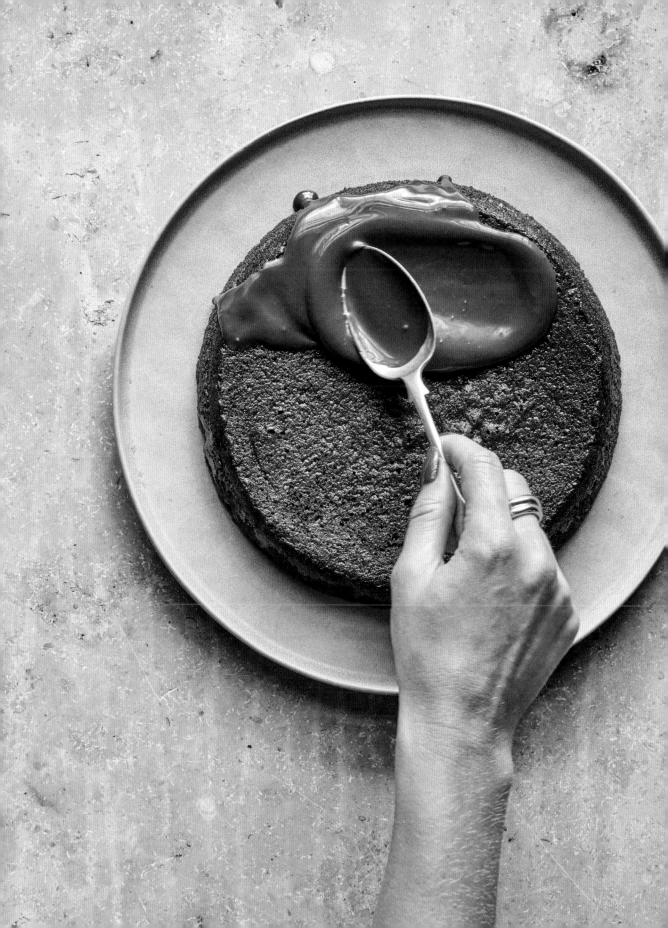

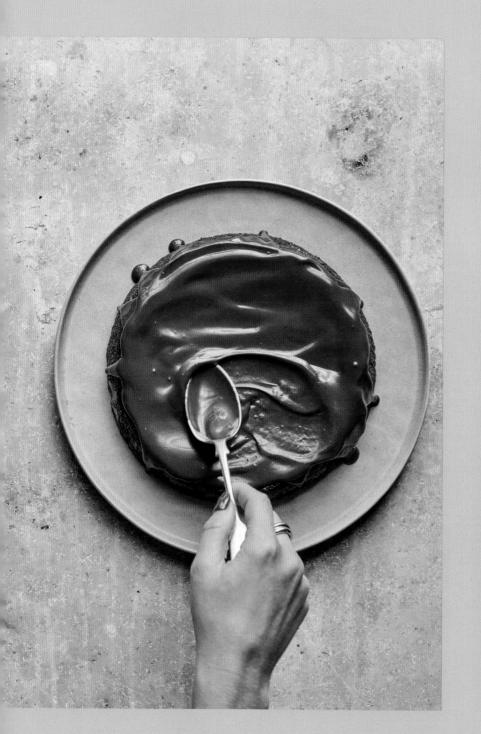
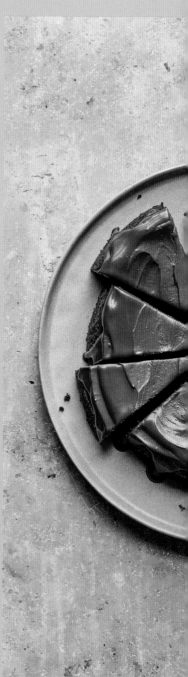

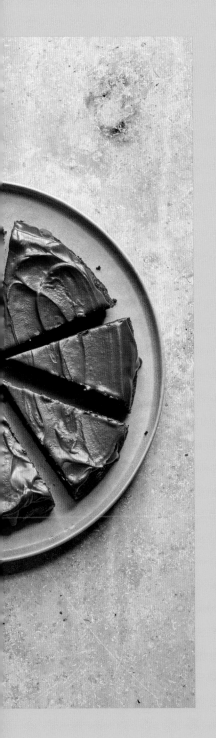
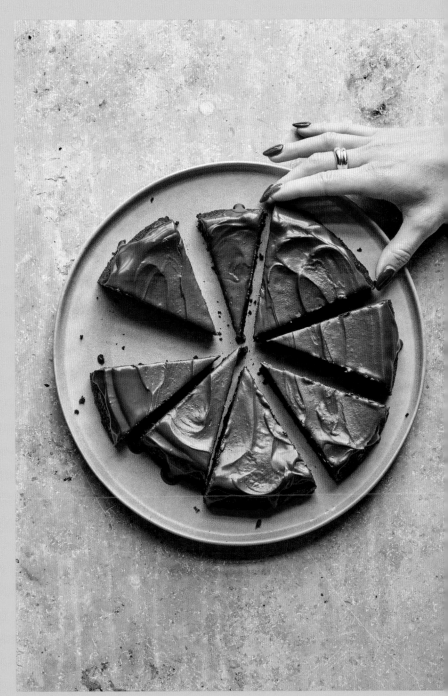

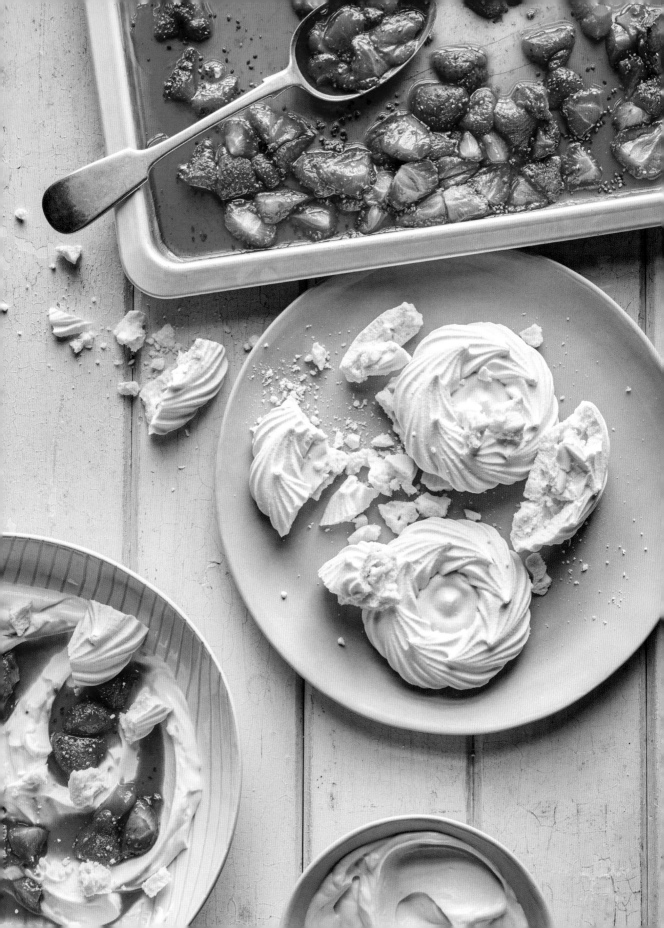

Greek Yogurt Roasted Strawberry Eton Mess

Serves 4

Time:
40 minutes, plus
cooling time

Macros:
Under 300kcal,
25g protein per serving

I actually prefer a creamy tangy Greek yogurt to cream in my Eton mess, which I know sounds controversial but when paired with the natural sweetness of roasted strawberries, the soft crunch of meringue and honey, it's just the most gorgeous dessert. This dish is high in protein from the yogurt, fibre-rich from the chia seeds and high in antioxidants from the strawberries, making it a delicious and nutritionally balanced treat.

500g (1lb 2oz) strawberries

2 teaspoons honey, plus an extra drizzle to finish

1 teaspoon vanilla extract

1 tablespoon chia seeds

500g (2¼ cups) Greek yogurt

4 ready-made meringue nests, crushed

Sprig of mint, to decorate

- Preheat the oven to 210°C/190°C fan (410°F) Gas Mark 6½.

- Hull the strawberries, then cut in half, or in quarters if they are large. Place in an ovenproof dish in a single layer.

- Drizzle the honey and vanilla extract over the strawberries, and sprinkle over the chia seeds. Mix gently to coat evenly.

- Roast the strawberries in the oven for 20 minutes, stirring occasionally, until they are starting to soften and release their juices, then remove and set aside to cool.

- In a serving bowl, begin layering the dessert. Start with some roasted strawberries, making sure you include some of the sticky cooking juices. Follow with a good dollop or two of yogurt and a sprinkling of crushed meringue.

- Repeat the layers, ending with strawberries, a drizzle of honey, and a touch of fresh mint to decorate.

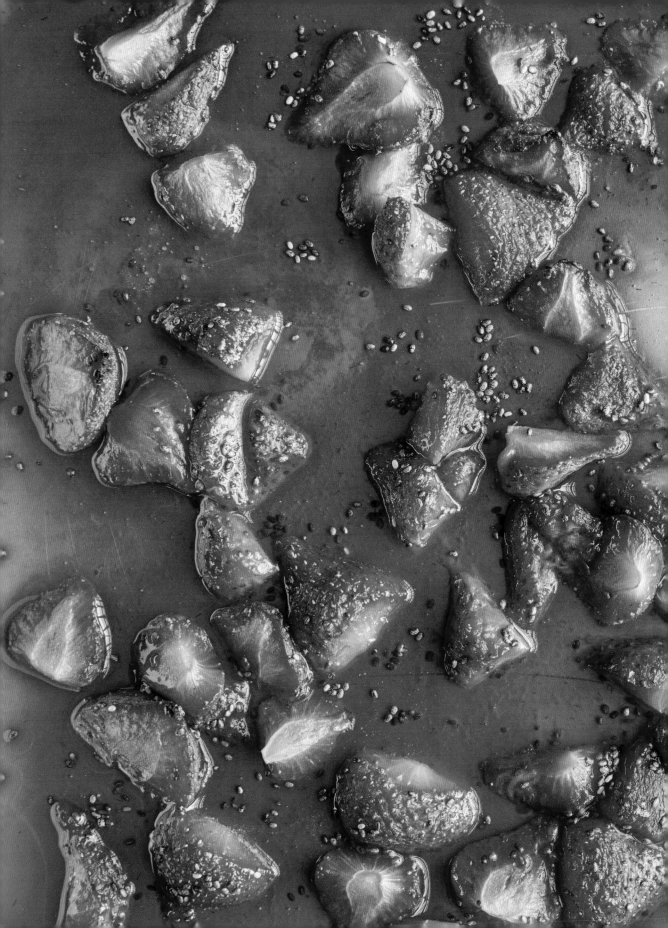

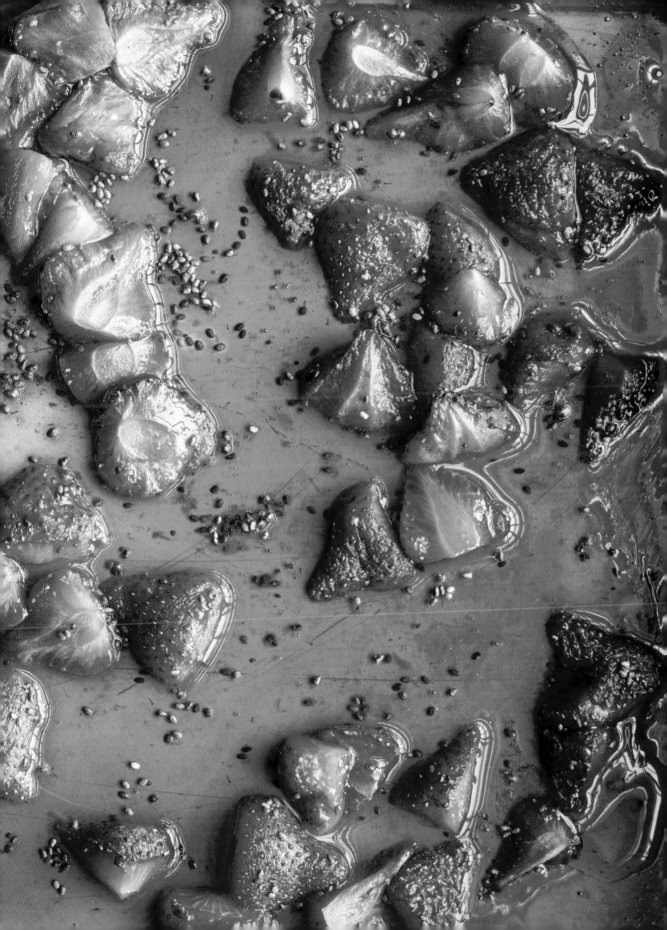

High Fibre Apple and Berry Crumble

A crumble is one of my go-to desserts, often making an appearance on a Sunday after a roast. It's so simple to throw together and wonderfully balanced to satisfy any sweet tooth, leaving you feeling wonderful. Fibre-rich apples and berries form the base, while the crumble is made with whole oats, almond butter and blood-sugar-stabilizing cinnamon. Pair with ice cream or custard – or, if you are like me, both!

Serves 6

Time:
50 minutes

Macros:
Under 300kcal,
4g protein per serving

400g (14oz) frozen mixed berries

2 Granny Smith apples, peeled, cored and diced

1 teaspoon chia seeds

Sweetener, e.g. stevia or honey to taste (optional)

For the crumble topping

2 tablespoons soft light brown sugar

200g (1½ cups) rolled oats

25g (scant 2 tablespoons) butter, cubed

2 tablespoons almond butter

1 tablespoon honey

1 teaspoon ground cinnamon

- Preheat the oven to 200°C/180°C fan (400°F) Gas Mark 6.

- In a saucepan, combine the frozen berries and diced apples. Cook over a medium heat for about 10 minutes, allowing the fruits to release their juices and soften. Stir in the chia seeds, remove from the heat and allow to cool slightly. Taste the fruit mixture: if desired, sweeten with a sweetener of choice.

- Meanwhile, in a bowl, prepare the crumble topping. Combine the sugar, oats, butter, almond butter, honey and cinnamon. Use your fingertips to rub the ingredients together until the mixture forms sticky clusters.

- Transfer the berry and apple mixture to an ovenproof dish. Evenly sprinkle the oat crumble over the fruit and then bake in the oven for 25–30 minutes, until golden brown.

- Serve warm with ice cream or custard. You can store your crumble in an airtight container in the refrigerator for up to 3 days, and enjoy either chilled or reheated.

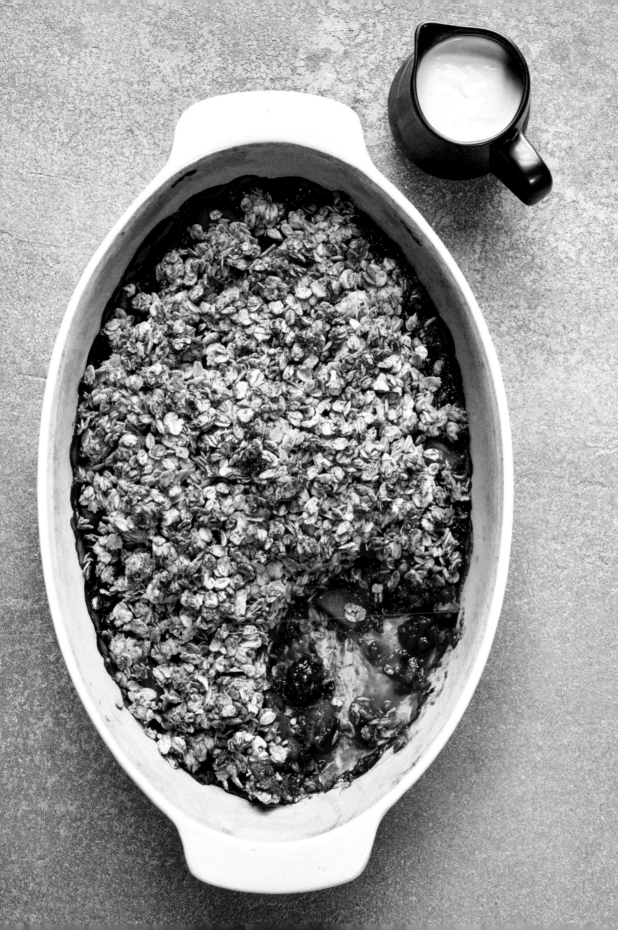

Bitter Lemon Tart

I love a super-lemony lemon tart and this Bitter Lemon Tart is just that. It offers a delicate balance of sweet and zesty, with the addition of half-fat crème fraîche bringing a welcome tangy richness. Ideal for days when you're after something refreshing yet fulfilling, it will keep in an airtight container in the refrigerator for up to 3 days. Top with fresh raspberries and go for another slice.

Serves 8

Time:
1 hour 15 minutes, plus cooling time

Macros:
Under 250kcal,
4g protein per serving

320g (11¼oz) ready-rolled shortcrust pastry (pie dough)

Plain (all-purpose) flour, for dusting

Raspberries, to serve

Icing (confectioners') sugar, for dusting

For the filling

3 medium free-range eggs, plus 2 free-range egg whites

40g (generous ¼ cup) icing (confectioners') sugar

2 tablespoons lemon zest (from about 4 unwaxed lemons)

150ml (⅔ cup) lemon juice (from 5–6 lemons)

200ml (scant 1 cup) half-fat crème fraîche

- Preheat the oven to 200°C/180°C fan (400°F) Gas Mark 6. Bring the pastry to room temperature about 20 minutes before using. Remove it from the packaging and unroll, keeping the provided nonstick baking paper.

- On a lightly floured surface, roll the pastry slightly thinner and cut out a circle to snugly fit a 20cm (8 inch) loose-bottomed tart tin (pan). Press any overhanging pastry down the sides of the tin. Dust with a little icing sugar to sweeten.

- Line the inside of the pastry with nonstick baking paper, fill with baking beans (pie weights) and blind bake in the oven for 20 minutes. Remove the beans and baking paper and return to the oven to bake for a further 5 minutes, until the base is golden and crisp.

- Remove from the oven and set aside to cool. Reduce the oven temperature to 150°C/130°C fan (300°F) Gas Mark 2. Once the pastry case is fully cooled, trim any overhanging edges with a serrated knife to achieve a neat finish.

- Meanwhile, make the filling. In a bowl, whisk together the eggs and egg whites in a gentle manner to prevent incorporating excessive air. Sift the icing sugar into a separate bowl, then gradually add the beaten eggs. Stir in the lemon zest and juice.

- In another bowl, beat the crème fraîche until smooth. Stir it into the lemon mixture, then transfer to a jug (pitcher) to ease the pouring process.

- Positioning the oven shelf halfway out, place your tart on it and delicately pour in the filling. Slide the shelf back in and bake for 25–30 minutes, until there is just a subtle wobble in the centre. Remove from the oven and leave the tart to cool for about an hour.

- Serve each slice topped with a raspberries and a dusting of icing sugar, if desired.

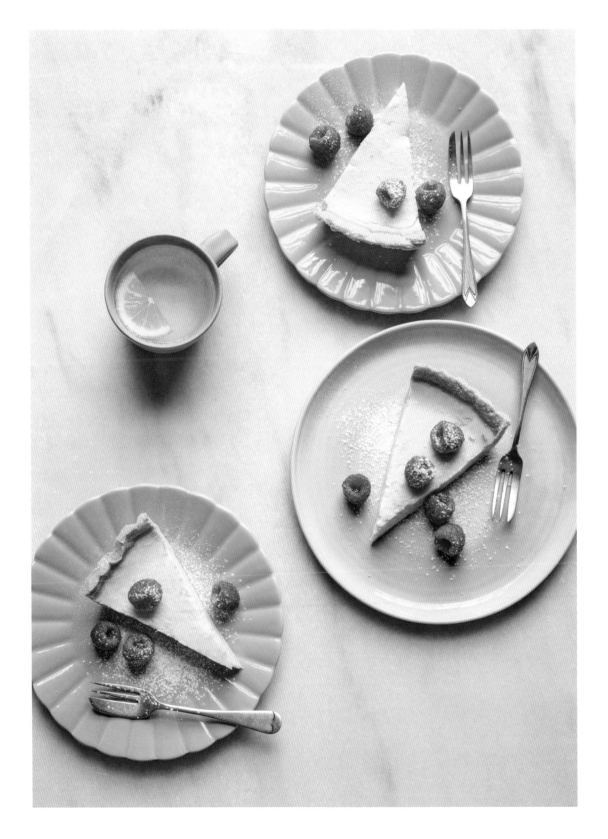

Victoria Sponge

Reinventing a classic, this ultimate celebration Victoria sponge is a timeless cake with a health-conscious spin. Infused with the zest and juice of a whole lemon, protein-packed natural yogurt and olive oil, it's moist, fluffy and quite simply divine. This cake celebrates the nostalgia of the traditional while embracing a more balanced approach – perfect for any occasion where indulgence meets a little hint of wellness. It can be stored in an airtight container in the refrigerator for up to 3 days.

Serves 12

Time:
1 hour, plus cooling time

Macros:
Under 350kcal,
3g protein per serving

Butter, for greasing

Zest and juice of 1 large unwaxed lemon

150g (¾ cup) caster (superfine) sugar

160g (⅔ cup) natural yogurt (low or 0% fat)

150ml (⅔ cup) olive oil

270g (2 cups) self-raising (self-rising) flour

2 large free-range eggs

For the filling

100g (scant ½ cup) low-fat cream cheese

100g (½ cup) thick natural yogurt (0% fat) or skyr

4 tablespoons icing (confectioners') sugar, plus extra for dusting

1 teaspoon vanilla extract

125g (4½oz) raspberries, lightly crushed

5 tablespoons high-fruit-content/intense raspberry jam

- Preheat the oven to 180°C/160°C fan (350°F) Gas Mark 4. Grease a 20cm (8 inch) cake tin (pan) with butter and line the base with nonstick baking paper.

- Pour the lemon juice into a small bowl and mix in 1 tablespoon of the caster sugar. Set aside.

- In a larger bowl, combine the lemon zest with the remaining sugar, adding in the yogurt, olive oil, flour and eggs. Mix well using a wooden spoon for about 1 minute or until uniformly combined.

- Carefully pour the batter into your prepared cake tin, and then bake in the oven for about 55 minutes, or until the cake has risen and gives a springy feel to a gentle touch.

- Remove from the oven and place the tin on a wire rack. While the cake is still hot, evenly spoon over the lemon juice and sugar mixture, allowing it to permeate the cake. Leave to cool completely before inverting the cake onto a plate or stand.

- For the filling, whisk together the cream cheese, yogurt, icing sugar and vanilla extract in a medium bowl, ensuring a smooth consistency.

- Cut the cake in half horizontally. On one half of the cake, spread a generous layer of the filling mixture, followed by a scattering of the lightly crushed raspberries. On the opposite half, spread an even layer of the raspberry jam. Unite the two halves, pressing gently. Dust with icing sugar, then serve.

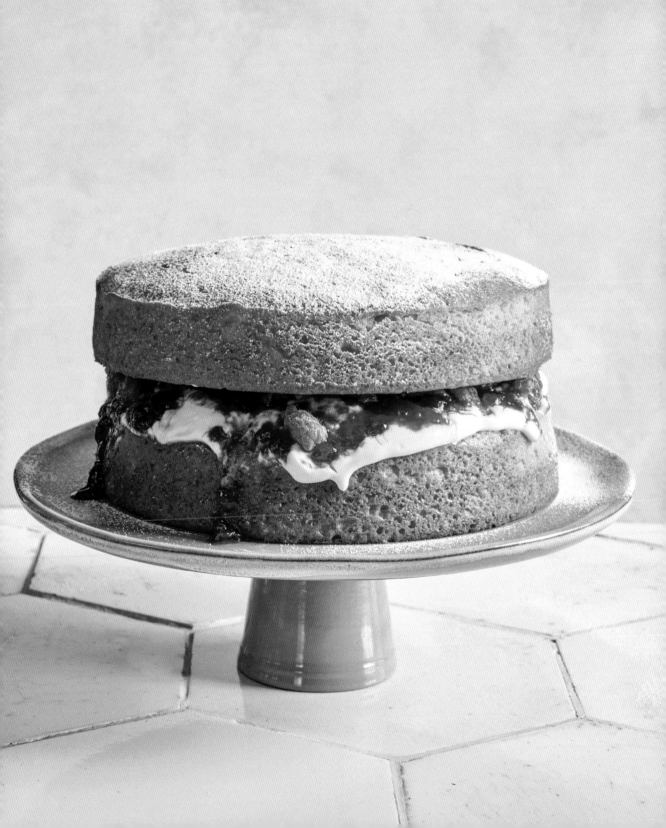

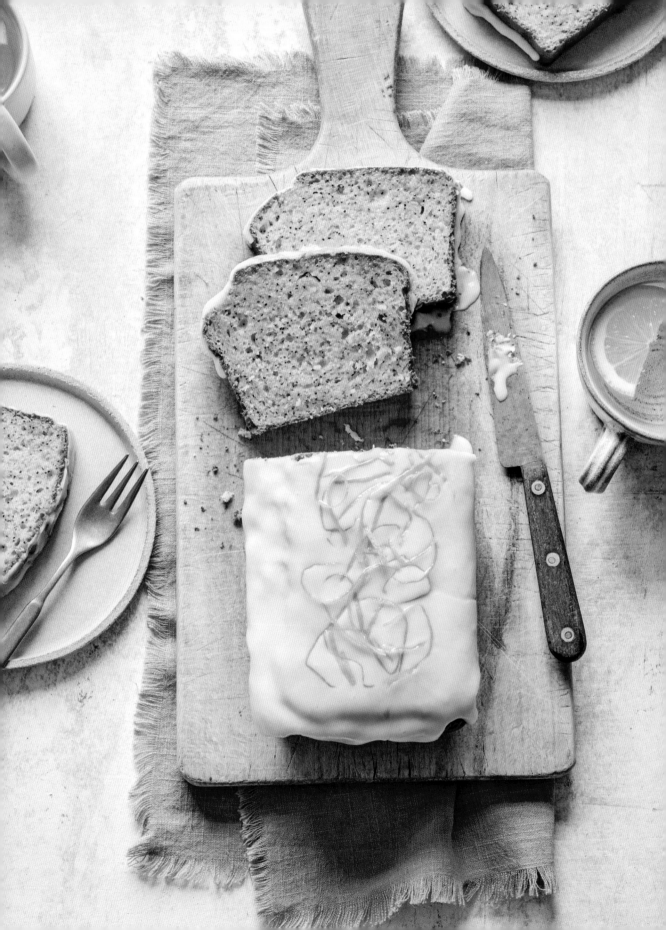

Gut Food Lemon Drizzle Loaf

Serves 10

Time:
1 hour 30 minutes,
plus cooling time

Macros:
Under 250kcal,
9g protein per serving

My spin on the classic lemon drizzle loaf cake, this recipe is packed full of gut-feeding fibre, healthy fats and balanced sugars, making this the perfect treat. Lemon drizzle was my favourite cake to make when growing up, and every time I bake this and the aroma of lemon fills my kitchen, it takes me straight back. Slice and serve with an extra dollop of natural yogurt, or store in an airtight container in the refrigerator for up to 5 days.

75ml (5 tablespoons) olive oil, plus extra for greasing

400g (2 cups) thick strained natural yogurt (0% fat) or skyr

1 teaspoon vanilla extract

Zest and juice of 2 unwaxed lemons, plus extra pared zest to finish

100g (½ cup) golden caster (superfine) sugar

2 large free-range eggs, at room temperature

100g (¾ cup) rolled oats, blended into a fine flour

100g (¾ cup) plain (all-purpose) flour

50g (½ cup) ground almonds

2 tablespoons poppy seeds

2 teaspoons baking powder

2 teaspoons bicarbonate of soda (baking soda)

For the drizzle

2 tablespoons honey

3 tablespoons lemon juice

For the icing (frosting)

50g (6 tablespoons) icing (confectioners') sugar

1 tablespoon lemon juice

- Preheat the oven to 180°C/160°C fan (350°F) Gas Mark 4. Grease a 900g (2lb) loaf tin (pan) with olive oil and line it with nonstick baking paper. If you are using a smaller tin, don't overfill or your cake will sink.

- In a bowl, combine the olive oil, yogurt, vanilla, lemon zest and juice, caster sugar and eggs until smooth. In another bowl, combine the oat flour, plain flour, ground almonds, poppy seeds, baking powder and bicarb, then gently fold it through the wet mixture until you have a smooth batter.

- Pour the batter into your prepared loaf tin, then bake in the oven for 1 hour or until golden brown and a cocktail stick (toothpick) inserted into the middle comes out clean. Set the cake to one side in the tin while you make the drizzle.

- In a small pan, warm the honey and lemon juice together until runny.

- Poke small holes all over the top of your cake using a toothpick and then spoon over the honey lemon drizzle evenly so it soaks into the cake. Allow to cool completely in the tin, then turn out onto a board.

- Mix together the icing ingredients until smooth but pourable. Spoon the icing over the top of your loaf cake, sprinkle extra pared lemon zest over the top, then serve.

194–199

Meal Plans

Meal Plans

WHEN YOU'RE MAKING MEAL PLANS, THINK ABOUT THE FOLLOWING:

- **Food Diversity:**
  Eating a variety of foods is essential for supporting our gut health. This meal plan shows you how to maximise food diversity to support your overall well-being.

- **Meal Prep:**
  Choose dinner recipes that can also serve as the next day's lunch to simplify meal prep and save time.

- **Oily Fish:**
  It is generally recommended to consume at least two portions of fish per week, of which at least one should be oily fish. Oily fish is high in omega-3 fatty acids, which are beneficial for heart health.

- **Protein Flexibility:**
  Feel free to swap proteins in recipes according to your preference. If a recipe calls for chicken, you're welcome to use another protein source to suit your preferences or swap in a high-protein legume or tofu to go veggie.

- **Cooking Flexibility:**
  You don't have to cook from scratch every day. Use the meal plan as a guideline for balancing your meals, and adjust as needed for your lifestyle.

I've left you some space to write out your own meals plans for the week, so you can tailor them to your preferences and lifestyle. Use these tips and the meal plan opposite as a basic guide to help you structure your main meals, and feel free to add in snacks or sweets to suit you.

Week 1

Monday
Breakfast: Prepable Breakfast Muffins
Lunch: Detox Gyoza Soup
Dinner: Chicken and Smoky Romesco
Snack Option: Romesco Dips

Tuesday
Breakfast: Prepable Breakfast Muffins (freeze leftovers if desired)
Lunch: Nature's Multivitamin
Dinner: Tuna Puttanesca Spaghetti

Wednesday
Breakfast: Chopped Egg Breakfast Toast
Lunch: Nature's Multivitamin (add protein)
Dinner: One-pan Tuscan Salmon

Thursday
Breakfast: Matcha Overnight Oats
Lunch: Speedy Chicken and Spicy Guacamole Tacos
Dinner: Creamy Coconut Thai Green Noodles

Friday
Breakfast: Eggy Bread with Tomato Salsa
Lunch: Sushi Salad
Dinner: Creamy Parmesan Chickpeas with Pickled Chilli (add protein)

Saturday
Breakfast: Fluffy Ricotta Lemon Pancakes
Lunch: Oven-baked Feta and Pepper Pasta
Dinner: My Best Ever Chicken and Tarragon Lasagne

Sunday
Breakfast: Lighter Sausage Breakfast Bagels
Lunch: Sticky Honey Halloumi Salad
Dinner: Superfood Vegetarian Bolognese

Sunday Notes: Consider batch cooking on weekends for easier meal prep during hectic days.

Week 2

Monday
Breakfast: Morning Tacos
Lunch: Mango, Jalapeño and Lime Salad
Dinner: Fish Pie with Garlic and Parmesan Crumb

Tuesday
Breakfast: Nutty Granola Clusters (pair with high-protein yogurt. Use leftovers as healthy snack ideas)
Lunch: Lighter Pesto Pasta Salad
Dinner: Spinach and Ricotta Malfatti

Wednesday
Breakfast: Pan con Tomate
Lunch: Crunchy Peanut Slaw
Dinner: Garlic-crumbed Salmon with Courgettes and Yogurt

Thursday
Breakfast: Tomato and Ricotta Breakfast Bowls
Lunch: Tuna Melt
Dinner: Thai Chicken and Butternut Soup

Friday
Breakfast: Chocolate Orange Oats with Citrus Honey
Lunch: Greek Salad-inspired Chicken Pittas
Dinner: Wholegrain Fish and Chips with Tartare Sauce

Saturday
Breakfast: Hot Honey Halloumi Avocado Toast
Lunch: Best Ever Caesar Salad
Dinner: Italian Sausage and Broccoli Pasta

Sunday
Breakfast: Sun-dried Tomato Shakshuka
Lunch: The Glow Bowl
Dinner: My Best Ever Chicken and Tarragon Lasagne

	Monday	**Tuesday**	**Wednesday**
Breakfast			
Lunch			
Dinner			
Snacks			

Thursday	Friday	Saturday	Sunday

	Monday	**Tuesday**	**Wednesday**
Breakfast			
Lunch			
Dinner			
Snacks			

Thursday	Friday	Saturday	Sunday

Colour Over Calories

This section is grounded in the principle that the nutritional value of food goes beyond just its caloric content. As a nutritionist, my aim is to guide you towards making informed choices about the foods you eat, emphasising the importance of a diverse and colourful diet.

The colours of fruits and vegetables are not just for show; they represent a wide range of essential nutrients and phytochemicals. Each colour group provides unique health benefits: red foods are often rich in antioxidants like lycopene, green vegetables are packed with chlorophyll and vitamins, while purple and blue foods are known for their anthocyanins, which support brain health.

I've shared my favourite foods in each of the colour categories, providing a straightforward way to ensure you're getting a broad spectrum of nutrients. Incorporating a variety of colours in your diet is a simple strategy to enhance your health, reduce disease risk and ensure you're getting the vitamins, minerals and antioxidants your body needs.

Let's focus on making our plates as colourful as possible, not just for visual appeal but for the health benefits this simple approach offers.

RED FOODS

- Examples: Tomatoes, red peppers, strawberries, raspberries, watermelon, red apples
- Key nutrient: Lycopene and vitamin C
- Benefits: Lycopene is a powerful antioxidant that's scientifically proven to help reduce the risk of certain types of cancer. It can also support heart health by reducing cholesterol levels and lowering blood pressure.

ORANGE FOODS

- Examples: Carrots, sweet potatoes, pumpkins, butternut squash, apricots, oranges, mangoes
- Key nutrient: Beta-carotene
- Benefits: Beta-carotene is converted to vitamin A in the body, which is essential for immune function, eye health and skin health. It also acts as an antioxidant to fight cell-damaging free radicals and is particularly important during the summer months.

GREEN FOODS

- Examples: Spinach, kale, broccoli, avocados, peas, chard, green apples, kiwis, salad leaves
- Key nutrient: Chlorophyll, folate, lutein
- Benefits: Green vegetables are rich in chlorophyll, which may have cancer-fighting properties. Folate is crucial for DNA synthesis and repair, while lutein supports eye health by protecting us against sunlight damage and reducing the risk of cataracts and age-related macular degeneration.

PURPLE/BLUE FOODS

- Examples: Blueberries, purple grapes, aubergines, beetroot, plums, purple sprouting broccoli, pomegranates, red cabbage
- Key nutrient: Anthocyanins
- Benefits: Anthocyanins have antioxidant properties that protect cells from damage and may reduce the risk of heart disease, stroke and cancer. They also improve memory and support healthy ageing.

YELLOW FOODS

- Examples: Bananas, yellow peppers, pineapples, yellow courgettes, lemons
- Key nutrient: Vitamin C and flavonoids
- Benefits: Yellow foods are often high in vitamin C, which supports the immune system, skin health and iron absorption. Flavonoids have antioxidant properties that can protect against chronic disease.

WHITE FOODS

- Examples: Garlic, leeks, onions
- Key nutrient: Allicin
- Benefits: While white foods aren't really 'coloured', it's worth mentioning that they contain allicin, which has antimicrobial and anti-inflammatory properties.

204-211

Index &
Conversions

Index

almonds
  chicken brick 105
  dark chocolate bites 95
  lemon drizzle cake 191
  & orange cake 173
anchovies 111, 126, 152
apple & berry crumble 184–5
avocado
  chicken & spicy guacamole tacos 52–3
  the glow bowl 67
  & Greek salad chicken pittas 75
  mango, jalapeño & lime salad 42
  in morning tacos 35
  sesame & ginger chicken salad 50
  speedy tuna salad 70–1
  sushi salad 62
  toast with feta eggs 38
  toast with hot honey halloumi 32–3

banana
  blueberry breakfast oat bars 7
  breakfast loaf 16–17
  oaty date banoffee pie 168–9
  in smoothie bowl 11
batch cooking xiii, xxi
beans, black 124
beans, butter 121, 122
beans, cannellini 85
beans, French 139, 163
beef & ricotta meatballs al forno 122–3
beetroot & mint dip 84, 86
berry & apple crumble 184–5
blueberries
  breakfast oat bars 6–7
  chia seed compote 9
  in smoothie bowl 11
bok choy, detox gyoza soup 58
Bolognese sauce, veggie 132–3
bread-based dishes
  avocado toast with hot honey halloumi 32–3
  chopped egg breakfast toast 18–19
  egg 'not-mayo' sandwich 69
  eggy bread with tomato salsa 30

English breakfast muffins 36
  Greek salad & chicken pittas 74–5
  pan con tomate 26
  Parmesan croutons 146–8
  prawn & sriracha burger 100
  sausage breakfast bagels 22
  tuna melt 46
  whipped feta & smoked salmon sandwich 64–5
breakfast xii
broccoli
  & Italian sausage pasta 152
  salmon & sexy veg 126
  sticky peanut stir fry 118
  Thai green noodles 130
bulgur wheat, glow bowl 67
burgers, prawn & sriracha 100
butternut squash
  & chicken Thai soup 156
  the glow bowl 67
  mac and cheese 98–9

cabbage, in slaws 48–9, 105
Caesar salad 56–7
cake
  banana bread loaf 16–17
  dark chocolate & olive oil torte 176–9
  lemon drizzle 190–1
  orange almond 172–5
  Victoria sponge 188–9
calories xiv
capers xx, 4
  feta & pepper pasta 72
  feta & smoked salmon sandwich 64
  multivitamin salad 55
  salmon & sexy veg 126
  speedy tuna salad 70–1
  tartare sauce 143
  tuna puttanesca spaghetti 111
carbohydrates xiv
carrots
  burger garnish 100
  chicken & tarragon lasagne 106
  creamy Parmesan chickpeas 150
  detox gyoza soup 58
  sticky peanut stir fry 118
  Thai green noodles 130
  in tomato soup 146
  vegetable Bolognese 132

cashew nuts 12
celery 132, 150
Cheddar cheese
   béchamel sauce 106
   breakfast bagels 22
   breakfast muffin fritatta 36
   mac and cheese 99
   tuna melt 46
chia seeds
   apple & berry crumble 184
   berry compote 9
   blueberry oat bars 7
   in Eton mess 181
   skin-glow crackers 88
chicken
   brick almond, with honey & lime slaw 104–5
   & butternut Thai soup 156
   the glow bowl 67
   & Greek-salad pittas 75
   & greens pot pie 114–15
   katsu curry 136–8
   nuggets with garlic yogurt 91, 92
   pesto pasta salad 61
   sausage & broccoli pasta 152
   sausage rolls 90, 93
   sesame & ginger salad 50
   and smoky Romesco 139–41
   & spicy guacamole tacos 52–3
   sticky peanut stir fry 118
   & tarragon lasagne 106–7
chickpeas
   creamy Parmesan, with chilli 150–1
   garlic-crumbed salmon 108
   hot & sour Thai bowl 163
   mango, jalapeño & lime salad 42–3
   multivitamin salad 55
   sesame & ginger chicken salad 50
   speedy tuna salad 70–1
   sticky halloumi salad 78
   see also hummus
chilli, pickled 150
chocolate
   almond bites 95
   & olive oil torte 176–9
coconut milk 130, 156
cooking methods xiv
cottage cheese 85
courgette (zucchini)

chicken & greens pot pie 114
chicken sausage rolls 90
chicken & tarragon lasagne 106
in fish pie 125
garlic-crumbed salmon 108
orzo 'ratatouille' 116
& prawn linguine 102–3
in ragù sauce 122
spiced turkey koftas 158
vegetable Bolognese 132
crackers/crispbread 86, 88, 89, 93
cream cheese 25, 188
crumble, oaty 184
cucumber
   burger garnish 100
   mango, jalapeño & lime salad 42
   multivitamin salad 55
   pickled 89, 136
   salad with salmon 68
   sesame & ginger chicken salad 50
   skin glow omega bowl 76
   speedy tuna salad 70–1
   sticky halloumi salad 78
   sushi salad 62
   in tabbouleh 158
   whipped feta & smoked salmon sandwich 64
curry
   chicken katsu 136–8
   Thai green 130

dates, banoffee pie 168
diet ix–x
   diversity ix, xiii, xvii
digestion xvii
dinner xiii
dips
   beetroot & mint 84, 86
   hummus 67, 84, 87
   pea & bean 85, 86

eggs
   bitter lemon tart 186
   breakfast muffin frittata 36
   in cakes 173, 176, 188, 191
   chopped egg toast 18–19
   crispy feta, with avocado toast 38–9
   eggy bread & tomato salsa 30
   English breakfast tray-bake 20–1

'not-mayo' sandwich 69
pan con tomate 26
ricotta & tomato breakfast bowl 4–5
scrambled, in tacos 35
with shakshuka 28–9
smoked salmon & cream cheese omelette 25
English breakfast tray-bake 20–1
equipment xviii-xix
Eton mess, strawberry 180–3

fats xiv
fermented foods xvii, xxi
feta
beetroot & mint dip 84
& chicken Greek-salad pittas 75
in chicken tacos 52
crispy feta eggs 38–9
garlic-crumbed salmon 108
the glow bowl 67
harissa red pepper soup 164
in morning tacos 35
multivitamin salad 55
orzo 'ratatouille' 116
& pepper pasta 72–3
with shakshuka 29
speedy tuna salad 70–1
whipped, smoked salmon sandwich 64
fibre ix, xii, xvii, xxi
filo pastry 90, 93
fish & chips, with tartare sauce 142–5
fish pie, with garlic & Parmesan crumb 125
flavour boosters xx
flaxseeds 88
food, processing xiv
frittata see eggs
frozen food xxi

garlic, roast 141, 146
gherkins, tartare sauce 143
glow bowl 66–7
grains xii, xx, xxi
granola clusters 12
gut health xvii
gyoza, detox soup 58–9

haddock, smoked, fish pie 125
halloumi 32–3, 78–9
harissa, red pepper soup 164

hazelnuts 12, 139, 176
hummus
caramelised onion 84, 87
the glow bowl 67

jalapeños 42, 52, 67

kale 114
katsu curry, chicken 136–8

leek
chicken & greens pot pie 114
chicken & tarragon lasagne 106
creamy 135
in fish pie 125
vegetable Bolognese 132
leftovers xiii
legumes, tinned xx
lemon
bitter lemon tart 186–7
lemon drizzle cake 190–1
Victoria sponge 188
lentils, in Bolognese 132
lettuce, Caesar salad 56
lifestyle xvii
linseed 88
lunch xii

mac and cheese, butternut squash 98
mackerel, smoked 76–7
macronutrients xiv
mango
jalapeño & lime salad with chickpeas & prawns 42–3
in smoothie bowl 11
matcha overnight oats 8
meatballs & ricotta al forno 122–3
meringue, yogurt & strawberry Eton mess 180–3
mint 84, 158
mozzarella 89
muffins, English, prepable 36
mushrooms
English breakfast tray-bake 20–1
vegetarian Bolognese 132

noodles, creamy coconut Thai green 130–1
nori sheets 62
nuts xx

oats xxi
  apple & berry crumble 184
  banana bread loaf 16
  banoffee pie base 168
  blueberry breakfast bars 7
  chocolate orange, with citrus honey 14–15
  lemon drizzle cake 191
  matcha overnight 8
  nutty granola clusters 12–13
  peach cobbler 170
olive oil xx
olives xx, 72, 111, 116
omelette *see* eggs
onions
  caramelised onion hummus 84
  red, pickled 52, 67
  in shakshuka 29
  see also spring onions
orange
  & almond cake 173
  chocolate orange oats 15
orzo 'ratatouille' & sea bass 116

pan con tomate 26
pancakes, ricotta lemon 2–3
pantry essentials xx-xxi
Parma ham 21, 56
Parmesan cheese
  chicken & greens pot pie 114
  chicken & tarragon lasagne 106
  chickpeas with chilli 150–1
  croutons 146–8
  fish pie crumb 125
  & harissa toast 164
  Italian sausage & broccoli pasta 152
  mac and cheese 99
  meatballs al forno 122
  pesto prawn courgetti linguine 102
  spinach & ricotta malfatti 129
  tuna puttanesca spaghetti 111
pasta
  baked feta & pepper 72–3
  butternut squash mac and cheese 98
  chicken & tarragon lasagne 106–7
  Italian sausage & broccoli 152–5
  orzo 'ratatouille', with sea bass 116
  pesto salad 60–1
  prawn & courgette linguine 102–3

tuna puttanesca spaghetti 111
  see also noodles
peach cobbler 170–1
peanut butter
  blueberry oat bars 7
  nutty granola clusters 12
  peach cobbler 170
  prawn & sriracha burger 100
  satay salmon 68
  sticky peanut stir fry 118
peanuts 49, 163
peas
  chicken & greens pot pie 114
  with fish & chips 143
  pea & bean dip 85
  sesame & ginger chicken salad 50
  sugar snap, peanut slaw 49
  sushi salad 62
pepperoni pizza crispbread 89, 93
peppers, red
  breakfast muffin frittata 36
  chicken & smoky Romesco 139
  chicken & tarragon lasagne 106
  creamy coconut Thai green noodles 130
  crunchy peanut slaw 49
  & feta pasta 72–3
  & harissa soup 164–5
  multivitamin salad 55
  orzo 'ratatouille' 116
  in ragù sauce 122
  in shakshuka 29
  smoky Mexican black bean soup 124
  sticky peanut stir fry 118
  Thai chicken & butternut soup 156
peppers, yellow 72–3, 116
pesto pasta salad 60–1
pitta bread, Greek-salad & chicken 74–5
plant-based foods xvii
pomegranate seeds
  the glow bowl 67
  multivitamin salad 55
  sticky halloumi salad 78
  in tabbouleh 158
poppy seeds 191
potatoes
  fish & chips 142–5
  mash 125
  salad, in omega bowl 76

prawns
    & courgette linguine 102–3
    in fish pie 125
    frozen xxi
    the glow bowl 67
    mango, jalapeño & lime salad 42–3
    pesto pasta salad 61
    & sriracha burgers 100–1
processed foods xiv
protein ix, xii, xiv
    long-lasting xxi
    powder 8, 11, 15
puff pastry 114, 135
pumpkin seeds 12, 55, 88

quinoa
    crunchy peanut slaw 49
    the glow bowl 67
    multivitamin salad 55
    sesame & ginger chicken salad 50
    in tabbouleh 158

radishes, pickled 50, 62
raspberries
    chia seed compote 9
    frozen raspberry 'popcorn' yogurt pot 94
    in smoothie bowl 11
    Victoria sponge 188
rice, brown xx
    chicken katsu curry 136
    chicken & smoky Romesco 139
    crunchy peanut slaw 49
    the glow bowl 67
    sticky peanut stir fry 118
    sushi salad 62
rice cakes 94
ricotta
    lemon pancakes 2–3
    in meatballs al forno 122
    & spinach malfatti 129
    & tomato breakfast bowl 4–5

salads
    Caesar 56–7
    crunchy peanut slaw 48–9
    cucumber, with salmon 68
    the glow bowl 66–7
    hot & sour Thai bowl 162–3

mango, jalapeño & lime with chickpeas & prawns 42–3
nature's multivitamin 54–5
pesto pasta 60–1
sesame & ginger chicken 50
skin glow omega bowl 76–7
speedy tuna 70–1
sticky honey halloumi 78–9
sushi 62–3
salmon
    creamy coconut Thai green noodles 130–1
    en croûte, with leeks 134–5
    in fish pie 125
    garlic-crumbed, courgettes & yogurt 108–9
    one-pot Tuscan 120–1
    satay, & cucumber salad 68
    & sexy veg 126–7
salmon, smoked
    & cream cheese omelette 25
    skin glow omega bowl 76
    & whipped feta sandwich 64
sauce
    béchamel 106
    Bolognese 132–3
    ragù 122
    Romesco 139–41
    tartare 143
sausage rolls, chicken 90, 93
sausages
    breakfast bagels 22–3
    & broccoli pasta 152
    English breakfast tray-bake 20–1
scallions see spring onions
sea bass, with orzo 116–17
seeds xx, 12, 86, 88
sesame seeds 88
shallots 102, 125, 139
shakshuka, sun-dried tomato 28
shortcrust pastry 186–7
smoothie bowl 10–11
snacks, mid-morning xii
soup
    detox gyoza 58–9
    harissa red pepper 164–5
    Mexican black bean 124
    roasted tomato with Parmesan croutons 146–9
    Thai chicken & butternut 156–7
spinach

breakfast bagels 22
in fish pie 125
one-pot Tuscan salmon 121
Parmesan chickpeas 150
& ricotta malfatti 129
skin glow omega bowl 76
smoked salmon & cream cheese omelette 25
sponge cake 188–9
spring onions
crunchy peanut slaw 49
garlic-crumbed salmon 108
skin glow omega bowl 76
sticky peanut stir fry 118
sushi salad 62
Thai green noodles 130
stir fry, sticky peanut 118
storecupboard foods xx–xxi
strawberry & yogurt Eton mess 180–3
stress xvii
sunflower seeds 12, 88, 168
sushi salad 62–3
sweet potatoes 78, 163

tabbouleh 158–9
tacos
chicken & guacamole 52–3
morning 34–5
tahini 78, 84, 168
tart, bitter lemon 186–7
Thai recipes
chicken & butternut soup 156
creamy coconut noodles 130–1
hot & sour bowl 162–3
tinned foods xx, xxi
tofu xxi
the glow bowl 67
jalapeño, mango & lime salad 42
tomatoes
breakfast bagels 22
Caesar salad 56
chicken & tarragon lasagne 106
chopped egg toast 18–19
crispy feta eggs 38
English breakfast tray-bake 20–1
& Greek salad chicken pittas 75
hot & sour Thai bowl 163
Mexican black bean soup 124
in morning tacos 35

one-pot Tuscan salmon 121
orzo 'ratatouille' 116
pan con tomate 26
pepperoni pizza crispbread 89, 93
pesto pasta salad 61
prawn & courgette linguine 102
in ragù sauce 122
& ricotta breakfast bowl 4
roasted tomato soup with Parmesan croutons 146–9
salsa with eggy bread 30–1
shakshuka 28–9
speedy tuna salad 70–1
spinach & ricotta malfatti 129
sun-dried xx, 36, 102, 106, 121
in tabbouleh 158
tuna puttanesca spaghetti 111
vegetarian Bolognese 132
tortilla, morning tacos 35
tuna xxi
puttanesca spaghetti 111
speedy salad 70–1
sushi salad 62
tuna melt 46–7
turkey, koftas with tabbouleh & mint yogurt 158

vegetables
diversity xiii
frozen xxi
vinegar xxi

wholefoods xiv, xx, xxi

yogurt xxi
egg 'not-mayo' sandwich 69
frozen raspberry 'popcorn' yogurt pot 94
garlic 91, 92
garlic-crumbed salmon 108
lemon drizzle cake 191
matcha overnight oats 8
mint 158
skin glow omega bowl 76
in smoothie bowl 11
& strawberry Eton mess 180–3
tartare sauce 143
tuna melt 46
Victoria sponge 188

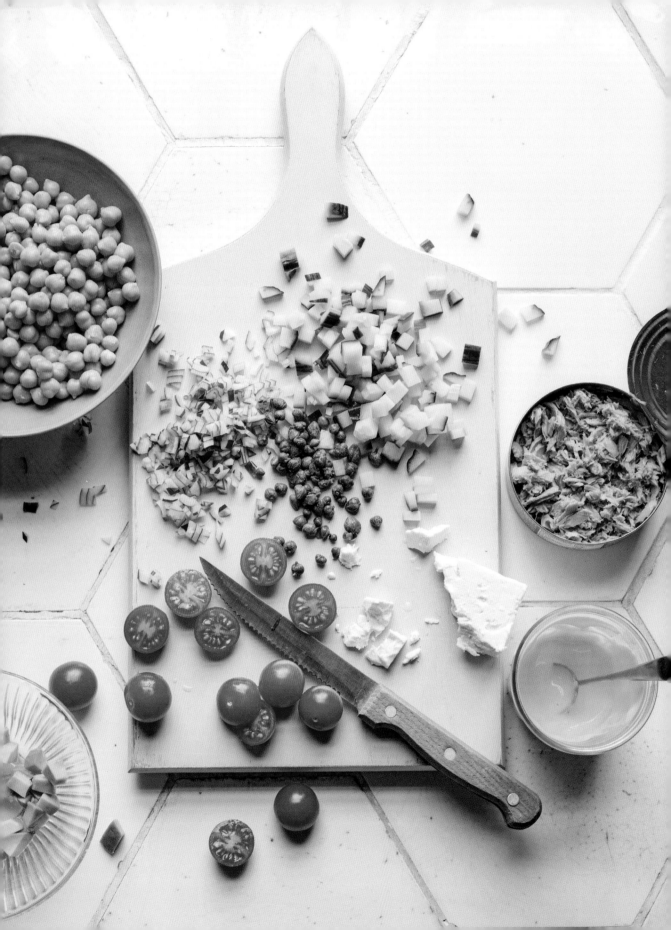

Conversions

Below are the main conversions for both metric and imperial units.
I have used metric scales when designing these recipes, so I recommend
following these quantities for the best accuracy.

WEIGHT CONVERSIONS

Grams	Ounces
10g	¼oz
15g	½oz
20g	¾oz
30g	1oz
40g	1½oz
50g	1¾oz
60g	2¼oz
70g	2½oz
80g	2¾oz
90g	3¼oz
100g	3½oz
150g	5½oz
200g	7oz
250g	9oz
300g	10½oz
350g	12oz
400g	14oz
450g	1lb
500g	1lb 2oz

VOLUME CONVERSIONS

Millilitres	Fluid Ounces
50ml	2fl oz
80ml	2¾fl oz
100ml	3½fl oz
125ml	4fl oz
150ml	5¼fl oz
175ml	6fl oz
200ml	7fl oz
225ml	8fl oz
250ml	9fl oz
275ml	9½fl oz
300ml	10½fl oz
350ml	12fl oz
400ml	14fl oz
500ml	18fl oz
750ml	26½fl oz
1 litre	35fl oz

LIQUIDS

Spoons & Cups	Millilitres
½ teaspoon	2.5ml
1 teaspoon	5ml
1 tablespoon	15ml
¼ cup	60ml
⅓ cup	80ml
½ cup	125ml
1 cup	250ml

Acknowledgements

I owe a huge thank you to several special people who have been instrumental in bringing this cookbook to life.

My Granny Janet, you sparked my initial fascination with cooking and restaurants, and I will always treasure the memories of spending Sundays working with you in the restaurant kitchen. Your signature recipes and passion for food will always continue to inspire me.

To my Nanny Mary, you showed me that food is more than nourishment; it's a way to express love.

To my mum, thank you for the countless home-cooked meals that brought comfort and stability to our busy family life. You have taught me the value of sharing meals with loved ones, you are all our rock.

And to Aaron, my partner. You've been there through every step of my journey, and I couldn't have done this without you. My biggest support and chief recipe taster.

Finally, to my editor George and the entire team behind the scenes at Orion. You have been instrumental in translating my vision of 'SO GOOD' into reality.

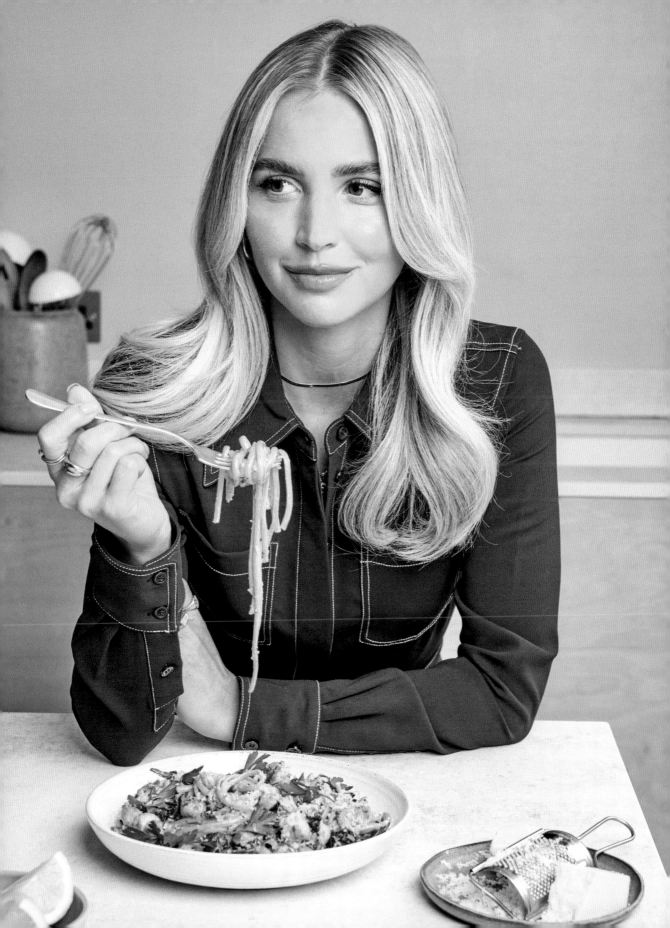

Credits

Publisher
Vicky Eribo

Commissioning Editor
George Brooker

Copy-editor
Sally Somers

Proofreader
Anne Sheasby

Indexer
Ingrid Lock

Editorial Management
Susie Bertinshaw
Jane Hughes
Charlie Panayiotou
Lucy Bilton
Claire Boyle

Contracts
Dan Herron
Ellie Bowker
Oliver Chacón

Art Direction
Helen Ewing

Designer
Nicandlou

Cover Design
Jessica Hart

Design
Nick Shah
Joanna Ridley
Natalie Dawkins

Photographer
Clare Winfield

Food and Props Stylist
Libby Silbermann

Food Stylist Assistant
Florence Blair

Production
Claire Keep
Katie Horrocks

Finance
Nick Gibson
Jasdip Nandra
Sue Baker
Tom Costello

Inventory
Jo Jacobs
Dan Stevens

Marketing
Helena Fouracre

Publicity
Ellen Turner

Sales
Jen Wilson
Victoria Laws
Esther Waters
Tolu Ayo-Ajala
Group Sales teams
across Digital, Field,
International, Non-Trade

Operations
Group Sales
Operations team

Rights
Rebecca Folland
Tara Hiatt
Ben Fowler
Alice Cottrell
Ruth Blakemore
Marie Henckel

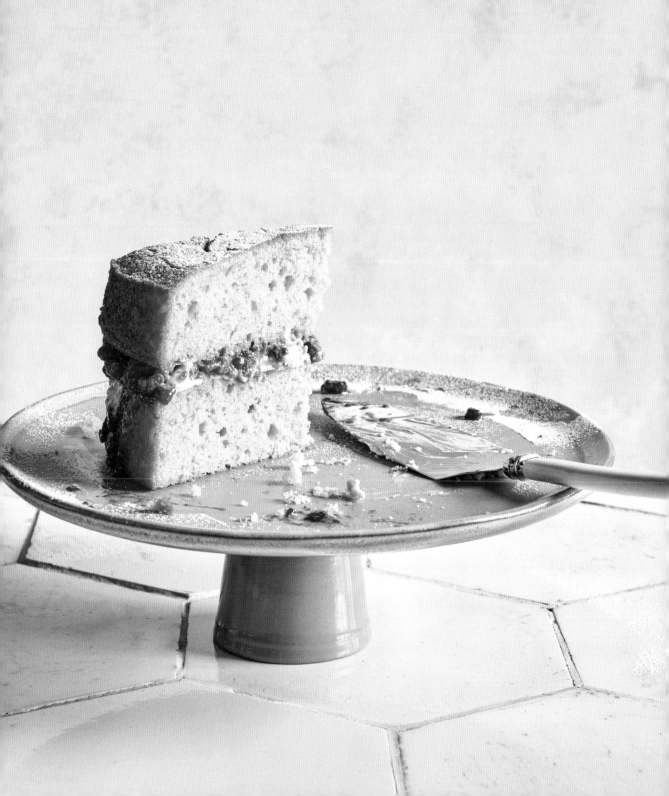

First published in Great Britain in 2024 by Seven Dials,
an imprint of The Orion Publishing Group Ltd
Carmelite House, 50 Victoria Embankment
London EC4Y 0DZ

An Hachette UK Company

9 10 8

A CIP catalogue record for this book is
available from the British Library.

ISBN (Hardback) 978 1 3996 2005 5
ISBN (eBook) 978 1 3996 2006 2

Typeset by nicandlou
Printed in the United Kingdom

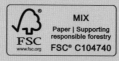

MIX
Paper | Supporting
responsible forestry
FSC® C104740

www.orionbooks.co.uk